LAUREN HELLIS

250 DELICIOUS AND WHOLESOME RECIPES

THE POTATO COOKBOOK

TABLE OF CONTENT

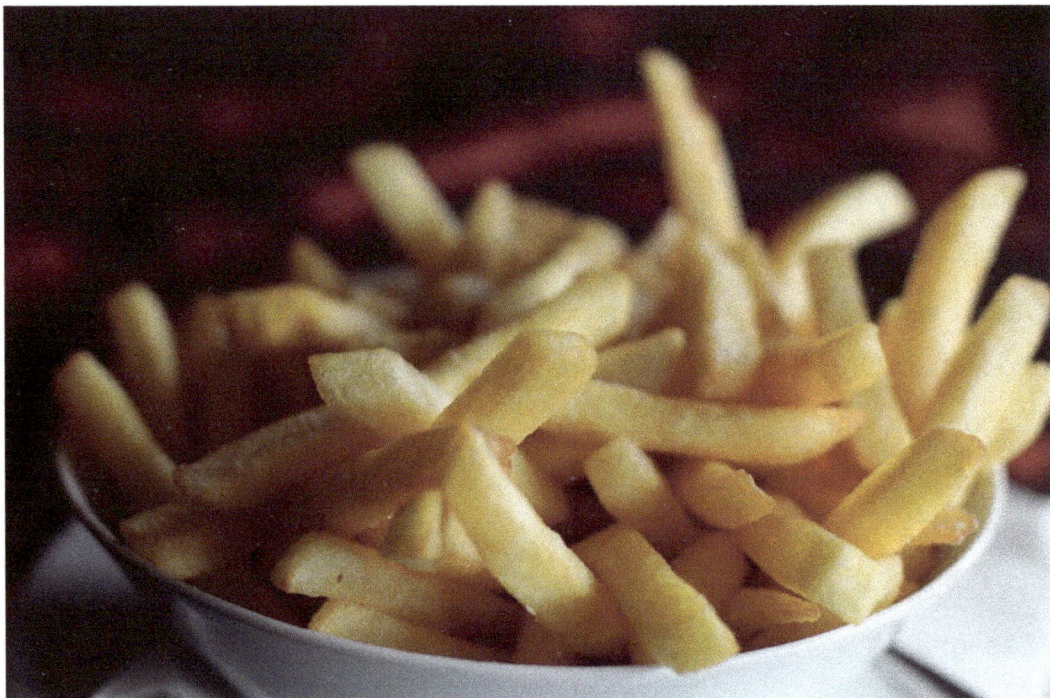

NUTRITIONAL VALUE OF POTATOES

Nutrients are classified as essential or nonessential. Essentialnutrients are obtained from food sourcesbecause the body does not produce them or produces them in amounts too small to maintain growth and health. Essentialnutrientsinclude water, proteins, fats, vitamins and minerals. Nonessentialnutrients are those manufactured by the body and do not need to be obtained from food, such as cholesterol.

Carbohydrates

Carbohydrates are the most abundant organiccompounds found in nature. They are produced by green plants and by bacteriausing the process known as photosynthesis, inwhichcarbondioxideis taken from the air by means of solar energy to yield the carbohydrates as well as all the other chemicals needed by the organisms to survive and grow. Carbohydrates are the human body's key source of energy, providing four calories of energy per gram (Smith 1988; Valdes 1998). When carbohydrates are broken down by the body, the sugar glucoseisproduced, whichiscritical to help maintaintissueprotein, metabolize fat, and fuel the central nervous system.

Potato carbohydrates may be classified as starch, non-starch, polysaccharides, and sugars. Starchis present in the form of granules, consisting of amylopectin and amylose in a fairlyconstantratio of 3:1. Amylopectinis a large, highlyramifiedmoleculecontaining about 105 glucoseresidues. The amylose moleculeis smaller, containing about 5000 glucoseresidues. There are small amounts of phosphorus, combinedchemicallywithstarch, mostly in the amylopectinfraction (Smith 1988).

When potatoes are subjected to heat duringcooking or processing, the water they containis absorbed into the starch granules, and the starchisgelatinized at temperatures of 70° C and above. The resulting gel usually remainsinside the potato cells unless these are ruptured duringcooking or other processing treatments such as mashing, inwhichcase the release of starch from the cells makes cooked potato very sticky (Smith 1988; Niederhauser 1993).

The highstarchcontent has made manufacture of potato starcheconomicallyfeasiblein developed countries. Potato starchis used in the manufacture of adhesives, in the textileindustry, in the food industry and for the production of derivedsubstancessuch as alcohol and glucose. Suchstarch gels set rapidly and has a high pot-paste viscosity, unlike those from cerealstarches (Smith 1988). The non-starchpolysaccharides are only a small part of the tuber dry matter. Non-starchpolysaccharides have an important role in the final texture of the cooked potato, becauseduringcooking the pectins are solubilized, and to some extent degraded, causingseparation, and occasionally rupture, of the cell walls. Non-starchpolysaccharidescontribute to the nutritional value of the potato because of itscharacteristic as dietaryfiber (Smith 1988; Niederhauser 1993).

The major sugars in the white potato are sucrose, fructose and glucose, although traces of some minor sugars are also found. Sugars are of considerableimportancein the potato flavor, and also ingiving a characteristiccolor to Frenchfries and chips (Smith 1988).

Lipids

The lipidcontent of potato is low. Galliard (1983) found 0.08 to 0.13% fresh weight bases in 23 varieties (Augustin et al. 1988). This range is too low to have any nutritionalsignificance but contributes toward potato flavor, enhances tuber cellularintegrity and resistance to bruising, and plays a part inreducingenzymicdarkeningin tuber flesh.

The greater importance of the lipidsliesintheirsusceptibility to enzymicdegradation and non-enzymic auto-oxidation, whichcause "off" flavor and rancidityin dehydrated and "instant" potato products. Galliard (1983) also has described the fatty acidcomposition of the lipid, and studied the lipid-degrading enzymes in 23 varieties of potatoes. He found that about 75 percent of the total fatty acids of the lipids are the polyunsaturated linoleic and linoleicacids.

These contribute to production of both desirable flavor characteristicsincooked tubers and undesirable "off" flavors inprocessedproducts. The polyunsaturated acids are rapidlyconverted to free fatty acids and other compounds by lipid-degrading enzymes during tuber processing, and are also extremely susceptible to auto-oxidation (Galliard 1983).ProteinsProteinis needed by humans, particularlyinfants, for growth, maintenance of tissues, restoration of losses caused by damage or disease, and pregnancy and lactation. Differentproportions of aminoacids are required for maintenance and for growth, and a particularprotein may be more effective for one purpose than for another (Smith 1988; Werge 1989).

Proteins are powerful compounds that build and repair body tissues, from hair and fingernails to muscles. Inaddition to maintaining the body's structure, proteins speed up chemicalreactionsin the body, serve as chemical messengers, fightinfection, and transport oxygen from the lungs to the body's tissues (Wolfe 1987; Smith 1988; Werge 1989). They are the predominantingredients of cells, making up more than 50 percent of the dry weight of humans. Humans have an estimated 30,000 differentproteins, of which only about two percent have been adequately described (Wolfe 1987). Although proteinsprovide four calories of energy per gram, the body uses protein for energy only ifcarbohydrates and fat intakeisinsufficient. When tapped as an energy source, proteinisdiverted from the many criticalfunctionsit performs in our bodies.

Proteins are made of smaller unitscalledaminoacids. Of the more than 20 aminoacids our bodiesrequire, eight (ninein some older adults and young children) cannot be made by the body insufficientquantities to maintain health. These aminoacids are consideredessential and must be obtained from food. Crude potato protein at about

2% fresh weightbasisiscomparable to that of most other root and tuber staples, with the exception of cassava, which has only half this amount. Itis also comparable, on a dry basis, with that of the cereals and, on a cookedbasis, with that of boiledrice (Werge 1989).

One advantage of the potato has over the cereal staples isitshighlysinecontent. However, itcontains lower concentrations of the sulfur-containingaminoacids, (such as methionine and cystine/cysteine) than the cereals. Incombinationwith other foods, potatoes can supplement diets that are limitinginlysine, such as riceaccompanying potatoes, whichprovides a better qualityprotein. In some developingcountries, meals are frequently served withmixtures of boiled potatoes and rice or pasta. However, suchmixtures are often wrongly assumed by developed-countryconsumers to providenothing more than large quantities of carbohydrate energy (Werge 1989).

It has been suggested that the comparative advantage of the potato as a foodstuff in the tropics, on a unitweightbasis, liesinitsability to supply high-qualityprotein. Using the latest figures for energy and proteinrequirements (FAO 1999), itcan be calculated that 100 grams (one small tuber) of potato can supply 7%, 6%, and 5% of the daily energy, and 12%, 11% and 10% of the dailyprotein needs of children aged 1-2, 2-3, and 3-5 years respectively. For adults, depending on body weight and sex, 100 grams of potatoes can supply from 3% to 6% of the dailyproteinrequirements. In a study in England in 1983, potato contributed 3.5% of the total household proteinintake. The proteincontribution of some other foods are the following: fruit, 1.3%, eggs, 4.6%, fish 4.8%, cheese 5.8%, beef 5.7%, white bread 9.8% and milk 14.6% (Werge 1989).

For infants and children, an energetically adequate dietcannot support growth ifitsproteincontentisinferior to the recommendeddailyrequirement. On the other hand, with an energeticallyinadequatediet, proteinismetabolized as an energy source, rather than being used for growth. Therefore, itisessential to consider the quality of a food or dietin terms of both protein and energy, for example, by the percentage of the total energy supplied by protein.

Regional food availability, costs, food preferences, preparationtimes, and cooking fuel costsmight also be considered on a localbasis when determining the relativeutility of the mixes. Potato requires less of the expensiveprotein-rich supplements than do other root, tuber and fruit staples, due to the highquality of itsprotein. (Werge 1989).

The only published work evaluating the quality of potato proteininfantdietsis that by Lopes de Romana et al. (1991) in Peru. Studieswithinfants and young childrenrecovering from malnutrition demonstrated that potatoes can supply all the dailydietaryrequirement of protein, and a substantial part of that for energy (Lopez de Romana et al. 1991).

Potato proteinis of sufficienthighquality for maintenance purposes in adult men, and for growth of infants and children. The relatively low digestibility of potato proteinis a disadvantage when potatoes are used for feedingchildrenbecause the potatoes have to be consumedin large quantities to satisfyprotein and energy requirements, a characteristic that potatoes share with other root and tuber staples. Potatoes are rarely consumed as the sole source of nitrogenin the diets of either adults or children, but they can make a valuable contribution to the proteincontent and the quality of a mixeddiet (Desborough and Lauer 1987). Plant breeders should not overlook the maintenance of protein levels in potatoes when searching for higher-yieldingvarieties.

Nitrogen

Potatoes are rarely eaten alone as the sole source of nitrogen and there are supplementary or synergisticeffects as a result of mixing potatoes with other foods. Potato is not a richsource of energy, supplyingapproximately 80 kilocalories per 100 grams, but itsupplieshigh-qualityprotein (Herrera 1989). Thisis of considerableimportanceindevelopingcountries, where energy supplies tend to be more readilyavailable than protein. The nitrogenouscontent of the potato tuber has a highnutritional value comparedwith many other vegetable crops, and there is a richliterature devoted to the subject.

Variationsin total nitrogen of potato tubers are attributable not only to differencesin the varieties, but also to cultivationpractices, climaticeffects, growing season, and location. The increase of total nitrogenwithincreasing levels of appliednitrogenis well-documented (International Potato Center 1991). Total nitrogen was increasedsignificantly also by applications of phosphorus of 56 kilograms per hectare. A study of the effects of moderate temperatures on tuber protein metabolism (22° C and 18 ° C for day and night, and 11° C and 7° C for day and night), showed that, in general, lower temperatures stimulated an increasein the percentage of tuber nitrogen. Marked differencesin total nitrogen were between varieties and between crops from different years and locations. Breeding-program selections for increase dnitrogen content should take place preferably inconditions representative of the intendedarea of production (International Potato Center 1991). Distribution of nitrogen within the tuber is not homogeneous (Herrera 1989), being highest in the skin, decreasingin the cortex and risingagain toward the pith. Desborough and Weiser (1974) reported that protein content was similarin the cortical, medullar and pithregions, while the pith area has significantly more non-protein nitrogen than the cortexti ssue (Ponnampalam and Mondy 1993).

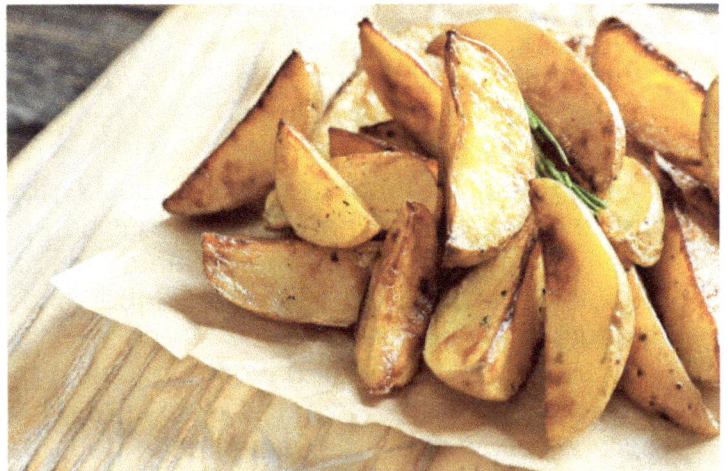

The total nitrogen of potato tubers includes: (a) soluble, coagulable (true) protein; (b) insoluble protein; and (c) soluble non-protein nitrogen, which is composed of free amino acids, the amides asparagine and glutamine, and small amounts of nitrate nitrogen and basic nitrogen compounds including nucleic acids and alkaloids. The insoluble protein fraction occurs mainly in the peel (Chang and Avery 1979). Itis only about four percent of total nitrogen. The proportion of soluble protein nitrogen to total nitrogen, considered to average about 50%, can range widely. A range of 29.5% to 51.2% was noted among 11 different S. tuberosum varieties, and of 40% to 74% in 50 clone samples of S. tuberosum group andigena (Bakel 1986).

There is a briefreview of adult human feeding experiments with potatoes by Knorr (1989). Incontrast to animal feeding trials, work with human adults has consistently shown that men or women can be maintainedinnitrogenequilibrium and good health on dietsinwhich all the nitrogen, or almost all, was supplied by potatoes (Knorr 1989). Herrera (1989) reported that Rose and Cooper (1917) maintained a young woman innitrogenbalance for seven days on an intake of 0.096 grams of nitrogen from potato per eachkilogram of body weight, and that Kon and Klein (1928) kept a man and a woman innitrogenequilibrium and good health for almost six months on a dietinwhich all the nitrogen required was supplied by potatoes.

The authors found that the daily need for potato protein was 36 grams for the man and 24 grams for the woman on a 70-kilogram body weightbasis (Herrera 1989). Kofranyi and Jekat (1987) are cited by various authors (Herrera 1989; Knorr 1989) as having determined that the average amount of proteinnecessary for the maintenance of nitrogenbalancein the case of three healthy college students was 0.545 grams per kilogram of body weight for potato, and 0.505 grams per kilogram of body weight for egg protein. Inaddition, the protein of potatoes has better nutritive value than the protein of beef, tuna fish, wheat flour, soybean, corn, beans or seaweed in terms of the quantitiesrequired to maintain nitrogen balance in adult human beings (Herrera 1989; Knorr 1989).

Amino acids

Aminoacids are an importantclass of organiccompounds. Of these, 20 serve as the buildingblock for proteins and as raw materials for the manufacture of many other cellularproducts, including hormones and pigments. Inaddition, several aminoacids are key intermediariesincellularmetabolism.

There are few completeaminoacid analyses of potato tubers in the literature. Kaldy and Markavis (1982) and Knorr (1989) provide tables of previous analyses by several authors, and report the aminoacidcompositions of several North Americanvarieties grown indifferentlocations. Knorr determined the aminoacidcompositions of potato samples withvarying levels of nitrogenintheir dry matter (Knorr 1989). The usual method of reporting tuber aminoacidcomposition has been used to evaluate the nutritive value of the potato. The proteinscores of six potato varietiesvaried from 60 to 78, on the basis of the sulfur-containingaminoacids (Kaldy and Markakis 1982).

The latest estimates of patterns of aminoacidrequirements for various age groups were published by FAO in 1999. Potato protein does not satisfy most of the aminoacidrequirements for infants, but has a very high average aminoacidscore of 90 for the pre-schoolchild, and scores of over 100 for all other age groups (Woolfe 1987). Potato protein has a particularly favorable lysine content in comparison with cereal proteins, whose aminoacidscores are much lower (Mudambi and Rajagopal 1990).

Concentrations of potato aminoacids have been reported in the literature, although there is a need for standardization to avoidconfusion, and to facilitatecomparisons of the nutritive value of the different samples. Meaningfulcomparisons of the capacity of different potato samples to satisfyprotein needs must be made on the basis of the aminoacidconcentrationsin the food as eaten, whichwill depend on the composition and on the content of tuber nitrogen (Kaldy and Markakis, 1982).

Enzymes

Enzymes are one of the many specializedorganicsubstances, composed of polymers of aminoacids that act as catalysts to regulate the speed of many chemicalreactionsinvolvedin the metabolism of livingorganisms. There are more than 700 enzymes identified, which are classified as hydrolytic, oxidizing, and reducing, depending on the type of reaction that they control (Valdes 1998). Hydrolytic enzymes acceleratereactionsinwhich a substanceis broken down intosimplercompounds through reactionwith water molecules. Oxidizing enzymes, known as oxidases, accelerate oxidation reactions; reducing enzymes speed up reductionreactions, inwhich oxygen is removed (Valdes 1998). Other enzymes catalyze other types of reactions.

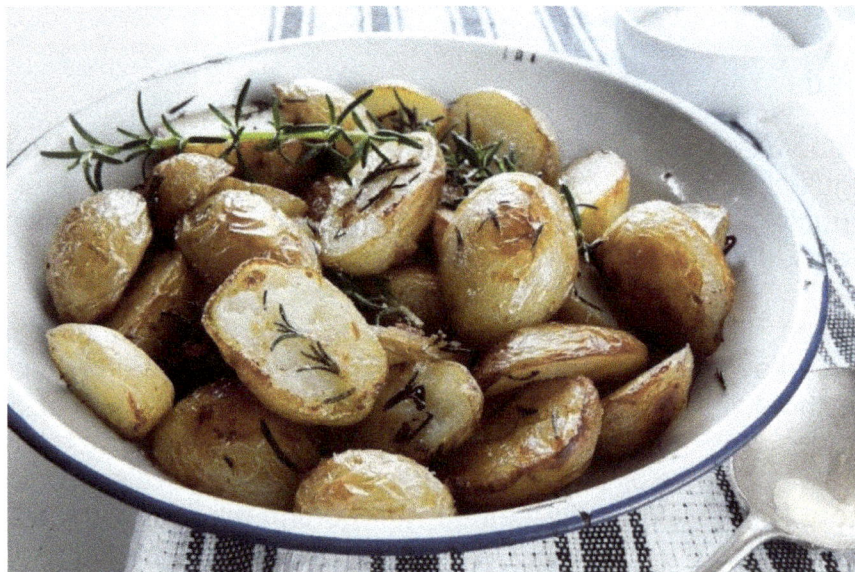

The potato contains numerous enzyme systems that constitute a considerableproportion of the total protein. The mechanism of low-temperature sweeteningduring storage occursbecause of the relativeactivities of enzymes and enzyme inhibitors (Linnemann et al. 1995). Phosphorylase (the action of which may be reduced by an inhibitor at higher temperatures) breaks down starch to glucose-1-phosphate. Some of thisisconverted to sucrose by sucrose phosphate synthetase (Linnemann et al. 1995).

Of the lipid-degrading enzymes, one is a lipolyticacyl hydrolase, whichliberates free fatty acids from phospholipids and glycolipids, and the other is a lipoxygenase that convertslinoleic and linolenicacids to their 9-hydroperoxide derivatives (Horton 1992). The importance of these enzymes in food processingistheir probable involvementin the formation of flavor and "off" flavor compounds (Horton 1992).

Another enzyme system, importantduring the preparation of both home-cooked and industriallyprocessed potatoes, causesenzymicdiscoloration or blackening of peeled or cut tubers. When tuber cells are injured, polyphenoloxidase (tyrosinase) gainsaccess to tyrosine and other orthodihydric phenols, which are oxidized to dark or

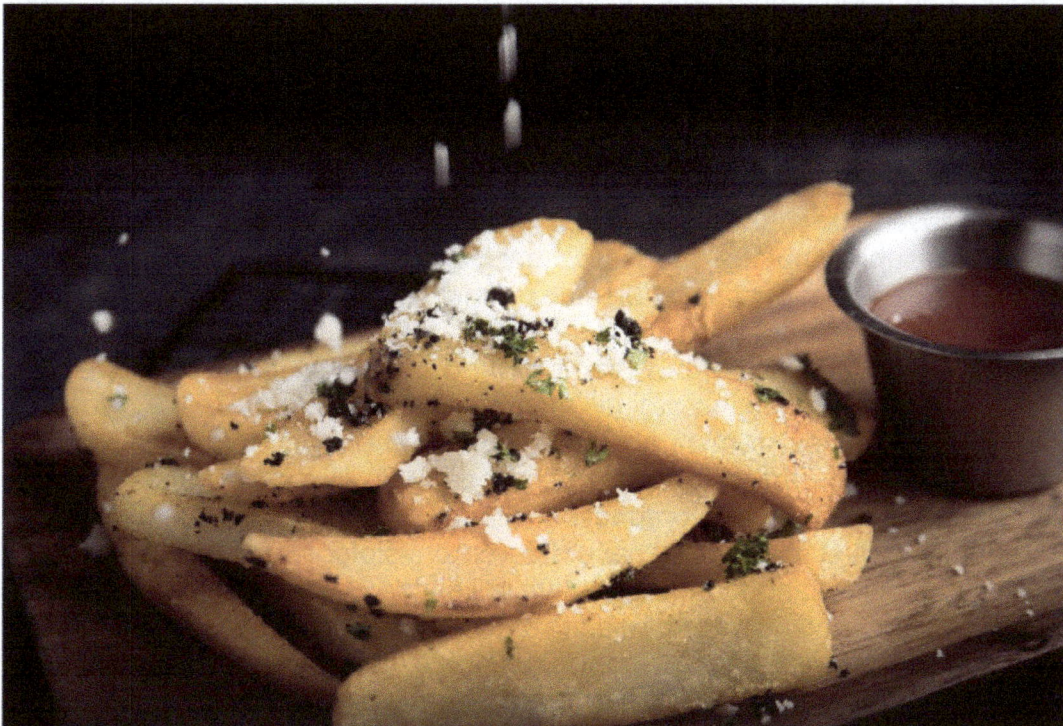

blackcompounds (melanins). Sincethisreactionisinitiated when cells are injured, some purchased potatoes may already have enzymicblackening as part of the flesh because of rough handling or mechanical damage.

This results in wastage when these tubers are prepared for cooking (or after cookinginskins), because the blackened parts are normally discarded. Also, high rates of enzymicdarkening are undesirable for industrialprocessingespecially for producers of pre-peeled potatoes. Smith (1988) brieflyreviewed the factorsaffecting the susceptibility of the potatoes to enzymicdiscoloration. These includedvariety, culturalpractices, and climaticconditions. The same author also reviewed the methods of inhibition of enzymic discoloration caused by peeling (Smith 1988).

Fiber

Inrecent years there has been increasing interest in dietary fiber, as a result of suggestions that it gives protection against divert iculosis, cardiovascular disease, coloncancer, and diabetes. Trowell (1960) defineddietaryfiber as "the plant polysaccharides and lignin that are resistant to hydrolysis by the digestive enzymes of man" (Liechsenring 1971). Dietaryfiberis not, however, a precise term, and opinions vary on its exact composition. Methods of determiningdietaryfiber are continually being modified and improved. Dietaryfiber analyses utilizephysiologicallyactive enzymes to break down non-fibercomponents, whileearlierchemicaldeterminations of crudefiber used acid or alkali. Crudefiber analyses have largely been abandoned because they measure only a small and variablefraction of the dietaryfiber (Liechsenring 1971).

Raw potato dietaryfibercontent ranges between one and two grams per 100 grams of fresh weight (Paul and Southgate 1988; Finglas and Faulks 1994). Inaddition, part of the dietaryfiber may be starch that isresistant to hydrolysis by the enzymes used to remove starchprior to dietaryfiberdetermination. This "resistantstarch" isproduced by subjecting the foods to heat or dehydration, whichconfers a more ordered structure on the starchmolecules, and renders them less susceptible to enzymatic digestion. Mudambi and Rajagopal (1990) found that there was little "resistantstarch" in raw potato, but that it formed from 20% to 50% by weight of the total dietaryfiber of cooked potato (Mudambi and Rajagopal 1990). However, itis unknown whether thisresistantstarchisdigestedin the human intestine. Ifitis not, then it should be considered part of the dietaryfiberbecause, like other types of fiber, may benefit health by helping the colonfunction (Mudambi and Rajagopal 1990).

Various types of dietaryfiber have differentphysiologicaleffects. Insoluble cereal fiber affects transittime and feca lweight, while soluble gel-formingfiberreduces serum cholesterol levels, and blood glucose and insulin response to meals contain ingcarbohydrates (Meuser and Smolnik 1989). A chemicalcharacterization of the dietaryfibersinvarious foods, including potatoes, revealed that cereal brans have the highestlignin values, are richinarabinoxylans and cellulose, but are low inuronicacids, whilevarious vegetables, including potatoes, have highercellulosecontent and more peptic and pectin-associatedsubstances than the brans. The significance of the findingsin terms of the nutritionalproperties of differentdietaryfibersources has not been determined (Meuser and Smolnik 1989).

Comparedwith other raw items, the fresh potato has dietaryfibercontentsimilar to sweet potatoes, but somewhat lower than that of other roots and tubers and much lower than most cereals and dry Phaseolus beans, although, on a dry basis, potatoes and content to soil type, location of growth, and the application of phosphorus (True et al. 1989).

Inaddition, there are great differencesin the contents of calcium, phosphorus, and ironin 13 varieties grown in the same location (Leichsenring et al. 1977). Wide ranges in some mineral elements, such as calcium, phosphorus, sodium, potassium, selenium and aluminum, were observed inninevarieties grown at fivelocations, and were attributed to location of growth rather than to variety. However, it was noted that these differencescould be due to other factors, including the mineralcontent of the soil, cultivationpractices or even samplingprocedures (Liechsenring et al. 1977).

Nitrogen fertilization had littleeffect on magnesium, calcium, potassium, sodium and phosphorus levels in "Russet Burbank" tubers, although the ironcontent was increased somewhat (Augustin 1985). Augustin also reported that potatoes grown on sandy soils had lower quantities of magnesium than those that were grown on loamy soils, but he concluded that the higherironcontentin tubers from sandy soil was a result of the ironcontent of the soil rather than of the soil type.

In potato, the ironcontentis about the same as in other roots and tubers, or some vegetables, and iscomparable on a dry weightbasis to cereals. Itishigher than the iron levels found inwhiterice, on either a dry or cookedbasis. Although not an outstandingsource of iron, 100 grams of cooked potatoes can supply between 6% and 12% of the dailyironrequirements for children or adult men (Smith 1988). The percentagecontributions are lower in women of child-bearing age, due to the greater demand for ironcaused by menstruation, pregnancy, and lactation.

The availability of iron may be enhanced by the presence of ascorbicacidingested at the same time as the ironsource. Potato ascorbicacidcontributes towards the level needed to influenceironabsorption from a meal. A positive correlation was found between the content of ascorbicacid of potatoes and the amount of ironsolubilized from potatoes by gastric juice invitro (Fairweather-Tait 1993).

However, a muchhigherproportion of the iron from potato was solubilizedinvitro than from other vegetable foods such as kidney beans, wheat flour and bread. It has been suggested that ironsolubilizationis the first step indeterminingironavailability from a food or meal. Therefore, potato appears to have a moderate ironavailability that issuperior to other vegetable foods (True et al. 1993; Fairweather-Tait 1993). In England, potatoes have been shown to supply 6% of the total household dietaryironintake, rankingthird of all individual foods as a dietarysource (Poats and Woolfe 1992). True et al. (1979) found that 160 grams of potato could supply from 2.3% to 19.3% of the United States recommendeddailyallowance (True et al. 1979). Thisrelatively large range is due to variationin the ironcontent found by the authors among varieties that were grown in several differentlocations. Also, it should be noted that the United States recommendeddailyallowance for ironisconsidered very high. If we use the more realisticrecommendeddailyallowancegiven by both FAO and WHO, potato makes a significantcontribution (True et al. 1979).

Potatoes are a good source of phosphorus, beingsimilar, inthisrespect, to roots and tubers and most cereals on a cookedbasis. Tortillas, bread and boiled P. vulgaris beans are richersources of phosphorus than potatoes. However, 100 grams of boiled potato supplies 7% of the United States recommendeddailyallowance for phosphorus for both children and adults (Quick and Li 1986).

A relatively small percentage of the total phosphorus in potatoes occursin the form of phyticacid. Phyticacidisinsoluble and cannot be absorbed in the human intestines. It also bindscalcium, iron, and zincin the form of phytates, rendering them unavailable for absorptioninto the body. About 25% of the total phosphorus was found in the form of phyticacidin seven commercial North American potato varieties (Quick and Li 1986).

The same authors quoted two sources that found that at least 80% of the phosphorus in potatoes was non-phytic (Swaminathan and Pushkarnath 1982). Incontrast, other plant foods containmuchhigher levels of phyticacid. In samples of field beans (Viciafaba), 40% to 60% of the total phosphorus was in the form of phytate phosphorus (Rhoades 1992). The lower phyticacidcontent of potatoes may be advantageous inallowing greater availability of the phosphorus, calcium, iron, and zincwhich may be present in a meal whichincludes potatoes.

Thisisespeciallyimportantin the case of calcium. Potato is a poor source of calcium, a characteristic that cooked potatoes share with other cooked staples, with the exception of lime-treated tortillas, P. vulgaris beans, and other legumes. With the exception of okra, no other vegetable is a particularly good source of calcium (Quick and Li 1986).

Magnesiumis another importantdietarymineral. For raw potatoes, 150 grams were found to provide between 6% and 10% of the United States recommendeddailyallowance for magnesium, and this range islikely to be the same for cooked potatoes, because there is almost 100% retention of the mineralin potatoes boiledintheirskin (Bretzloff 1981).

In the United States, recommendeddailyallowances have been established for only two of the trace elements found in potatoes: zinc and iodine. Comparingfigures for levels of zinc and iodinein potatoes with the United States recommendeddailyallowance levels, 100 grams of potato should provide 13% of adult, and up to 30% of childrequirements of iodine, and 2% and 4% of adult and childrequirementsrespectively of zinc. Labib (1982) has noted that biologicalavailability of zincis generally lower in vegetables than in foods derived from animals (Labib 1982).

Other, less extensivelyinvestigatedtrace elements reported to have beneficialeffectsin humans includecopper, chromium, manganese, selenium and molybdenum (Meikejohn 1973). It has been shown that 100 grams of potatoes can supply at least part of the dailyrequirement for copper, manganese, molybdenum and chromium (Labib 1982; Espinola 1989). True et al. (1989) found that a 150-gram serving of potatoes supplies 8% of the United States recommendeddailyallowance for cooper (True et al. 1989). The same authors determined that the manganese content of potatoes ranged from 0.7 to 1.9 mg/kg, and that it made a partialcontribution to the 15% of dailyintakeprovided by all fruits and vegetables in the Britishdiet. According to a study made by Spring et al. (1979), potatoes provided 10% of the magnesium, 11% of the copper and 3% of the zinc of the Britishdiet. A more recentanalysisrevised these contributions to 8.4% and 4.3% for copper and zinc, respectively (Finglas and Faulks 1994). Lastly, potatoes are not a good source of selenium, containing less than 0.01 mg/kg. (Espinola 1989)

Other trace elements, for which no requirements have been established, but inwhich some interest has been shown, includecobalt, nickel, fluoride, and vanadium. Potato is not an outstandingsource of fluoride and inthisrespectissimilar to most other foods (Davies 1987). The content of vanadiumis less than 1 ng/g (Joseph et al. 1983).

Organic acids

The major organicacidsidentifiedin the potato arecitric and malicacids. Other organicacids present in smaller amounts in the potato areoxalic and fumaric, chlorogenic and phosphoric as well as ascorbic, nicotinic, and phyticacids, aminoacids and fatty acids. All these contribute to flavor. The level of malicacidcan be used as an indication of tuber maturity. Ascorbicacid and nicotinic acids influence directly, and phytic acid indirectly, the nutritional value of the potato (Schwartz et al. 1982).

Chlorogeni cacid can react with ferric ions during cooking to produce a dark-coloredcomplex. This phenomenon, known as post-cooking or non-enzymaticblackening, may occur more in the "heel" than in the "rose" end of the potatoes, inwhichcaseitiscalled stem-end blackening. Citricacidsin tubers prevent this by sequestering the iron present and makingitunavailable for forming a complex with chlorogeni cacid. The susceptibility of potatoes to post-cookingblackening depends on the relative concentrations of iron and of chlorogenic and citricacids (Augustin et al. 1988).

Pigments

Potato flesh may be white or various shades of yellow, depending on the variety. Yellow colorationis generally due to the presence of carotenoidpigments. The major carotenoididentifiedin a study of 13 German varieties of potatoes was violaxanthin, followed by lutein and lutein-5, 6-epoxide, and, in lower concentrations, neoxanthin A and neoxantin. B-carotene was detected only intrace amounts or was totally absent (Augustin 1985). Anthocyaninpigmentsin the periderm and peripheralcortexproduce totally or partly pigmentedskinsin potatoes. In some South Americanvarieties, the pigmentis so dark that some tubers may appear black and others dark purple. Another type of pigmentationoccursbecause of chlorophyll.

When harvested, potato tubers exposed to light form chlorophyll forms in the superficial parts of the skin, givingit a green color (Augustin 1985). Very littleis known about the nutritional value of the different potato pigments (Woolfe 1997). Itispossible that, in some varieties, the yellow color may be due to other, unidentifiedpigments as well as to carotenoids. In some places, such as Peru, yellow-fleshed varieties of potatoes are highlyprized and commandhigherprices than potatoes withwhite flesh.

Vitamins

Among many other functions, vitaminsenhance the body's use of carbohydrates, proteins, and fats. They are criticalin the formation of blood cells, hormones, nervous system chemicals known as neurotransmitters, and the genetic material deoxyribonucleicacid (DNA). Vitamins are classifiedinto two groups: fat soluble, and water soluble. Fat-soluble vitamins, which include vitamins A, D, E, and K, are usually absorbed with the help of foods that contain fat. Fat containing these vitaminsis broken down by bile, a liquid released by the liver, and the body then absorbs the breakdown products and vitamins. Water-soluble vitamins, whichincludevitaminC (ascorbicacid), B1 (thiamine), B2 (riboflavin), B3 (niacin), B6, B12, and folicacid, cannot be stored and rapidly leave the body inurineif taken in greater quantities than the body can use (Page and Hanning 1983; Smith 1988; Valdes 1998). Foods that contain water soluble vitamins need to be eaten daily to replenish the body's needs.

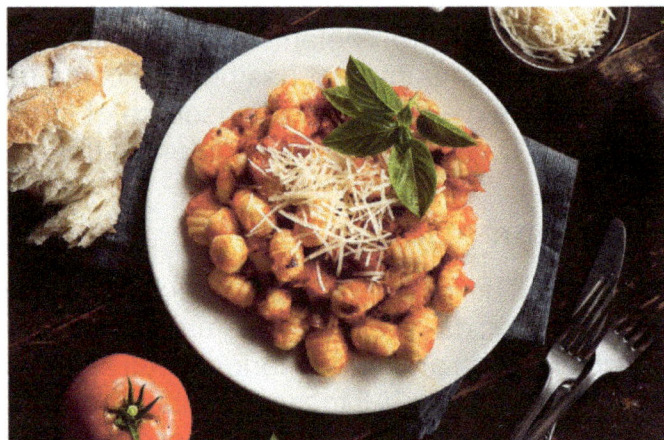

Potatoes are substantialsources of several vitamins: ascorbicacid (vitaminC), and the B vitamins: thiamin (B1), pyridoxine (B6), and niacin. Riboflavin (B2), folicacid and pantothenicacid are also present, as well as small amounts of vitamin E. Biotinis present only intraces (Meikejohn 1973). VitaminCexistsin the tuber in both the reduced and oxidized forms. In the freshly harvested raw tuber the reduced form L-ascorbicacidisquantitatively the most important, although dehydroascorbicacidis also present. In the stored, cooked or processed potatoes, only the L-ascorbicacidis generally present (Page and Hanning 1983). This vitamin is importantin the formation and maintenance of collagen, the protein that supports many body structures and plays a major role in the formation of bones and teeth. It also enhances the absorption of iron from foods of vegetable origin.

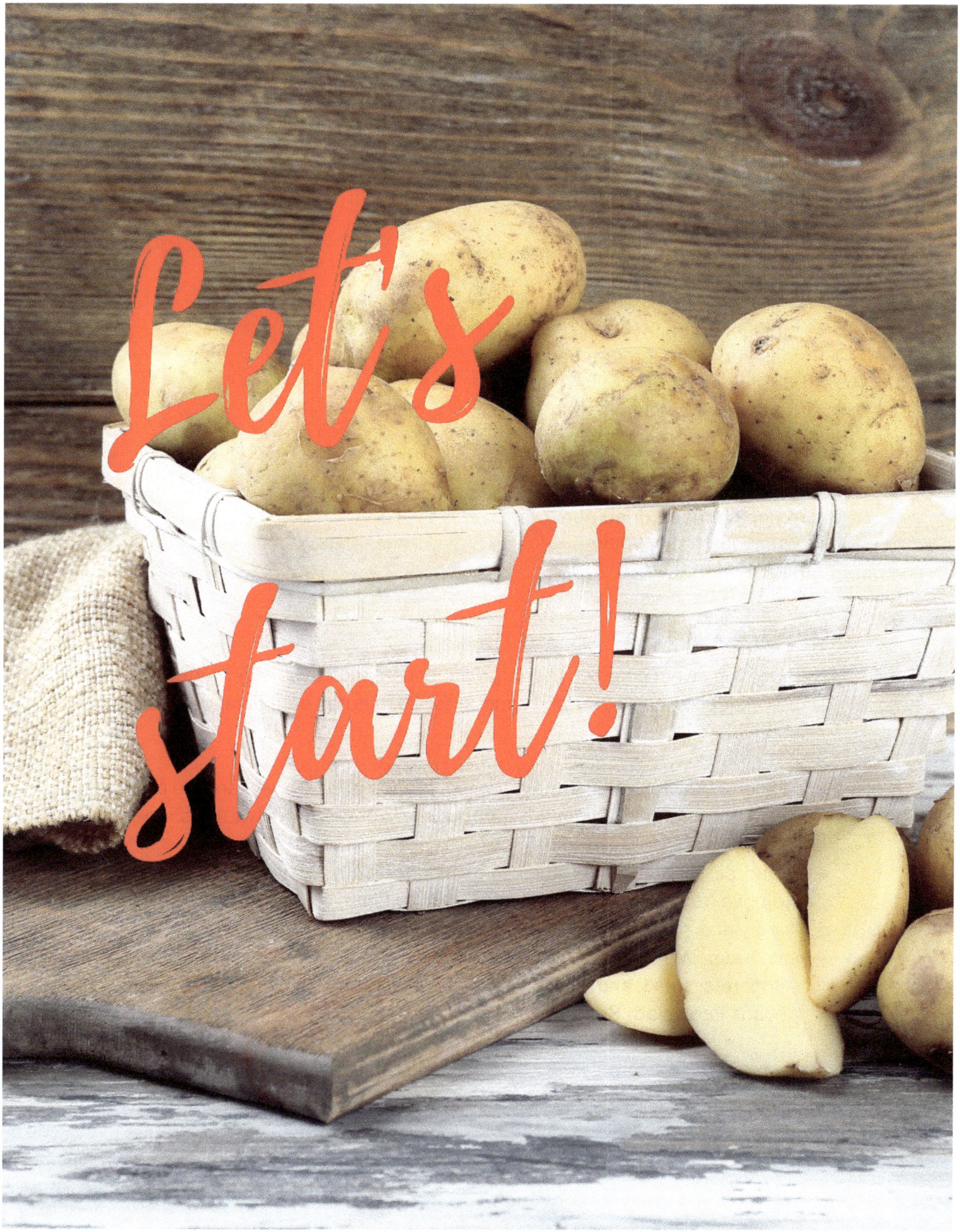

Let's start!

Ham and Sweet Potato Salad

Ingredients

- ❋ 4 cups cubed peeled sweet potatoes
- ❋ 1 cup mayonnaise
- ❋ 1/3 cup orange juice
- ❋ 1 tablespoon honey
- ❋ 1 tablespoon grated orange peel
- ❋ 1/8 teaspoon salt
- ❋ 1/8 teaspoon ground ginger
- ❋ 1/8 teaspoon ground nutmeg
- ❋ 1 1/2 cups julienned fully cooked ham
- ❋ 2 celery ribs, thinly sliced
- ❋ 1/4 cup chopped dried apricots
- ❋ 1 whole fresh pineapple
- ❋ 1 cup chopped pecans

Directions

➢ Place the sweet potatoes in a large saucepan and cover with water. Bring to a boil. Reduce heat; cover and simmer for 20 minutes or until tender. Drain and cool.

➢ In a large bowl, combithe mayonnaise, orange juice, honey, orange peel, salt, ginger and nutmeg. Stir in the ham, celery, apricots and sweet potatoes.

➢ Stand pineapple upright and cut in half vertically, leaving the top attached. Remove fruit, leaving a 1/2-in. shell. Cut fruit into chunks;

➢ stir 1 cup into the salad (save remaining fruit for another use). Cover and refrigerate salad and shells for at least 4 hours. Just before serving, stir pecans into salad. Spoon into pineapple shells.

Bacon Cheese Potatoes

Ingredients

- ❀ 8 medium potatoes
- ❀ 1/2 cup finely chopped onion
- ❀ 1 pound process American cheese, cubed
- ❀ 1 cup mayonnaise
- ❀ 1/2 pound sliced bacon, cooked and crumbled
- ❀ 3/4 cup sliced black olives
- ❀ Chopped fresh parsley Paprika

Directions

➢ Peel the potatoes; place in a saucepan and cover with water. Cook until tender but firm; drain and cube. In a bowl, mix potatoes with onion, cheese and mayonnaise.

➢ Transfer to an ungreased 13-in. x 9-in. x 2-in. baking dish. Sprinkle with bacon and olives. Cover and bake at 350 degrees F for 30 minutes or until heated through. If desired, sprinkle with parsley and paprika.

Skewered Grilled Potatoes

Ingredients

- 2 pounds red potatoes, quartered
- 1/2 cup water
- ½ cup light mayonnaise
- 1/4 cup dry white wine
- 2 teaspoons crushed dried rosemary
- 1 teaspoon garlic powder
  wooden skewers, soaked in water for 30 minutes

Directions

➤ Place potatoes and water in a microwave safe bowl. Cook potatoes in microwave on high until just tender, about 15 minutes, stirring half-way through.

➤ Drain potatoes and allow to steam for a few minutes to dry. In a large bowl, stir together mayonnaise, wine, rosemary, and garlic powder.

➤ Mix in drained potatoes and toss to coat. Marinate, covered, in the refrigerator for 1 hour.

➤ Preheat an outdoor grill for high heat and lightly oil grate. Remove potatoes from marinade, and skewer.

➤ Grill, covered, for 6 to 8 minutes, brushing occasionally with marinade, turning half-way through. Remove potatoes from skewers and serve hot.

Sweet Potato-Turkey Meatloaf

Ingredients

- 1 large sweet potato, peeled and cubed
- 1 pound ground turkey breast
- 1 large egg
- 1 small sweet onion, finely chopped
- 2 cloves garlic, minced
- 1/4 cup honey barbecue sauce
- 1/4 cup ketchup
- 2 tablespoons Dijon mustard
- 2 slices whole-wheat bread, torn into small crumbs
- 1 tablespoon freshly ground black pepper, or to taste
- 1 tablespoon salt, or to taste

Directions

➢ Preheat oven to 350 degrees F (175 degrees C). Lightly grease a 2 quart baking dish. Bring a pot of lightly salted water to a boil. Add the sweet potato, and cook until soft, about 10 minutes. Drain the sweet potatoes, and mash or whip until smooth.

➢ Mix the ground turkey together with the egg, sweet onion, garlic, barbecue sauce, ketchup, Dijon mustard, and whole wheat bread crumbs in a large mixing bowl. Season to taste with salt and pepper. Add the sweet potatoes, and stir until evenly combined.

➢ If the mixture seems too wet, add more bread crumbs. Use your hands to form the turkey mixture into a loaf shape and place in the prepared baking dish. Bake in the preheated oven 1 hour. Slice the loaf to serve.

Potato Pancakes I

Ingredients

- 4 large potatoes
- 1 yellow onion
- 1 egg, beaten
- 1 teaspoon salt
- 2 tablespoons all-purpose flour ground
- black pepper to taste
- 2 cups vegetable oil for frying

Directions

➢ Finely grate potatoes with onion into a large bowl. Drain off any excess liquid.Mix in egg, salt, and black pepper.

➢ Add enough flour to make mixture thick, about 2 to 4 tablespoons all together. Turn oven to low, about 200 degrees F (95 degrees C).

➢ Heat 1/4 inch oil in the bottom of a heavy skillet over medium high heat. Drop two or three 1/4 cup mounds into hot oil, and flatten to make 1/2 inch thick pancakes. Fry, turning once, until golden brown.

➢ Transfer to paper towel lined plates to drain, and keep warm in low oven until serving time. Repeat until all potato mixture is used.

Russian Potato Salad from Costa Rica

Ingredients

- ❁ 4 potatoes, peeled and cubed
- ❁ 1 (15 ounce) can sliced beets, drained and finely chopped
- ❁ 4 eggs
- ❁ 2 tablespoons mayonnaise, or as needed
- ❁ salt and pepper to taste

Directions

➢ Place the potatoes into a pot and cover with salted water. Bring to a boil over high heat, then reduce heat to medium-low, cover, and simmer until tender, about 20 minutes.

➢ Drain and allow to steam dry for a minute or two. Allow the potatoes to cool. While the potatoes are cooking, place the eggs into a saucepan in a single layer and fill with water to cover the eggs by 1 inch.

➢ Cover the saucepan and bring the water to a boil over high heat. Once the water is boiling, remove from the heat and let the eggs stand in the hot water for 15 minutes.

➢ Pour out the hot water, then cool the eggs under cold running water in the sink. Peel and dice once cold. Place the potatoes, beets, eggs, and mayonnaise into a bowl, mix well, and season to taste with salt and pepper.

Peppery Scalloped Potatoes

Ingredients

- 1 (10.75 ounce) can condensed cream of mushroom soup,
- undiluted
- 1 1/2 cups milk
- 1/2 teaspoon salt
- 1/8 teaspoon cayenne pepper
- 5 cups peeled and thinly sliced potatoes
- 1/4 cup butter or margarine, melted
- 1/4 cup all-purpose flour

Directions

- In a small bowl, combine the soup, milk, salt and cayenne; set aside. Place a third of the potatoes in a greased 13-in. x 9-in. x 2-in.

- baking dish; layer with a third of the butter, flour and soup mixture. Repeat layers twice. Bake, uncovered, at 350 degrees F for 1 hour and 20 minutes or until potatoes are tender.

Cheesy Potato Soup I

Ingredients

- 2 cups chicken broth
- 4 large potatoes, diced
- 2 stalks celery, chopped
- 2 carrots, chopped
- 1/2 onion, chopped
- 4 cups milk
- 12 (1 ounce) slices processed cheese food
- 1/4 cup dry potato flakes
- 4 slices crisp cooked bacon, crumbled

Directions

➢ In a large pot combine the chicken broth, potatoes, celery, carrots and onion. Mix together and bring to a boil over medium heat. Cook 15 to 20 minutes or until vegetables are tender.

➢ Add milk; reduce heat to medium low and let simmer. Add cheese slices; when cheese is melted, slowly stir in dry potato flakes until mixture is slightly thickened. Sprinkle bacon on top and serve hot.

Fourth of July Potato Salad

Ingredients

- ❀ 3 pounds potatoes, peeled and diced
- ❀ 1/3 cup cider vinegar
- ❀ 2 teaspoons white sugar
- ❀ 1 1/2 teaspoons dry mustard
- ❀ 1 1/2 teaspoons salt
- ❀ 3/4 teaspoon ground black pepper
- ❀ 1/2 cup mayonnaise
- ❀ 1/2 cup sour cream
- ❀ 1/4 cup heavy cream
- ❀ 3/4 cup chopped onion
- ❀ 3 hard-cooked eggs, peeled and chopped

Directions

➤ Bring a large pot of salted water to a boil, add the potatoes and let cook until tender. While the potatoes cook, in a large bowl, whisk together the vinegar, sugar, mustard, salt and pepper.

➤ Drain the potatoes, stir them into the vinegar mixture and let them marinate for 30 minutes to absorb the flavors.

➤ In a small bowl, whisk the mayonnaise, sour cream and heavy cream. Fold this creamy mixture into the potato mixture along with the onions and hard-cooked eggs.

➤ Cover and chill before serving if you wish. (This salad keeps for up to 3 days in the refrigerator.)

Southern Comfort Sweet Potatoes

Ingredients

- 2 (29 ounce) cans sweet potatoes, drained
- 1/2 cup butter, softened
- 1 teaspoon ground cinnamon
- 1/4 cup orange juice
- 3 eggs, beaten
- 1/4 teaspoon salt
- 1/2 cup Southern Comfort liqueur
- 1/2 cup chopped pecans
- 1/2 cup light brown sugar

Directions

➤ Preheat oven to 350 degrees F (175 degrees C). Place sweet potatoes in a large bowl. Beat with an electric mixer until light and fluffy. Mix in the butter, cinnamon, orange juice, eggs, salt, and liqueur.

➤ Transfer to a 2 quart casserole dish. Mix the pecans and brown sugar in a small bowl, and sprinkle evenly over the sweet potato mixture. Bake 30 to 40 minutes in the preheated oven, or until center is firm and edges are lightly browned.

Allana's Excellent Potato Soup

Ingredients

- 8 ounces cubed cooked ham
- 1 cup chopped onion
- 1 tablespoon butter
- 2 1/2 pounds potatoes, peeled and diced
- 2 (14.5 ounce) cans chicken broth
- 1 tablespoon prepared Dijon-style mustard
- 1 1/2 cups milk
- 1 (10.75 ounce) can condensed cream of celery soup
- 1/4 teaspoon garlic powder
- 1/4teaspoon seasoning salt
- 1/2teaspoon salt-free seasoning blend

Directions

> In a large saucepan over medium-high heat, sautee ham and onions in the butter, until the onions are translucent. Stir in the mustard,then pour in the chicken broth. Add potatoes, bring to a boil and cook until potatoes are tender.

> Combine the milk and cream of celery soup; stir in to the saucepan. Season with garlic powder, seasoned salt and salt-free seasoning blend. Heat through, but do not boil. Serve hot.

Potatoes in Paper

Ingredients

- 4 potatoes, sliced
- 4 small onions, sliced
- 4 tablespoons butter
- 4 slices Cheddar cheese
- 1 cup water

Directions

➤ Preheat oven to 350 degrees F (175 degrees C).Cut out 4 12x12 inch sheets of aluminum foil. Place one sliced potato, one sliced onion, 1 tablespoon butter and one slice of cheese on each aluminum foil square.

➤ Wrap the foil around the sides of the potatoes and onion to form a cup. Pour 1/4 cup of water into each pouch and fold the top of aluminum foil over the potatoes to close it.Bake in a preheated 350 degrees F (175 degrees C) oven for 60 minutes.

Sweet Potatoes for Two

Ingredients

- ❀ 2 sweet potatoes, cooked and peeled
- ❀ 1/2 cup packed brown sugar
- ❀ 2 tablespoons butter or margarine
- ❀ 2 tablespoons water
- ❀ 1/4 teaspoon salt
- ❀ 1 dash ground nutmeg or ground mace

Directions

➤ Slice sweet potatoes into an 8-in. pie plate; set aside. In a saucepan, combine brown sugar, butter, water and salt; bring to a boil.

➤ Pour hot syrup over potatoes. Bake, uncovered, at 350 degrees F for 30 minutes, basting occasionally, or until syrup thickens and potatoes are glazed. Sprinkle with nutmeg or mace.

Twice Baked Potatoes

Ingredients

- 4 large baking potatoes
- 1/2 pound bacon
- 4 tablespoons butter
- 1 large onion, chopped
- 1/2 cup chopped fresh mushrooms
- 1 teaspoon crushed red pepper
- 1 teaspoon garlic powder
- 1 teaspoon ground black pepper
- 1 teaspoon chopped fresh chives
- 1 teaspoon salt
- 1 (8 ounce) container sour cream
- 1 (8 ounce) package shredded Cheddar cheese
- 1 teaspoon dry bread crumbs

Directions

- Preheat oven to 400 degrees F (200 degrees C). Use a fork to pierce the potato skins.Bake the potatoes unwrapped for about 1 hour, or until soft, in the preheated oven.Place bacon in a large, deep skillet. Cook over medium high heat until evenly brown. Drain, crumble and set aside.

- Over medium-low heat melt the butter in a large saucepan. Combine onion, mushrooms, red pepper, garlic powder, pepper, chives and salt. Cook slowly, stirringoccasionally until the onions are soft.

- Slice open the baked potatoes and, keeping the skins intact, scoop the insides into a medium bowl. Transfer the onion mixture to the bowl. Mix in the sour cream. Pour in 1/2 of the cheese and continue mixing until all ingredients are well blended.

- Using a large spoon, fill the potato skins with the mixture. Top with bread crumbs, the remaining cheese and bacon.Return the potatoes to the preheated oven and continue baking for about 15 minutes, until the cheese is melted and the filling is slightly brown.

Honey-Topped Sweet Potato

Ingredients

- 1 small sweet potato
- 2 tablespoons butter or margarine, softened
- 4 teaspoons brown sugar
- 2 teaspoons honey
- 1/8 teaspoon ground cinnamon

Directions

➤ Wrap potato in foil; bake at 400 degrees F for 45-50 minutes or until soft when gently squeezed. In a bowl, combine the butter, brown sugar, honey and cinnamon until smooth.

➤ Cut an "X" on top of potato. Using a fork, fluff the pulp. Add the butter mixture; fluff with potato until melted.

Potato and Pork Bake

Ingredients

- 8 potatoes, cubed
- 8 thick cut pork chops
- 1 packet dry onion soup mix

Directions

➤ Preheat oven to 400 degrees F (200 degrees C).Place the potatoes in a 10x15 inch baking dish and arrange the pork chops over the potatoes. Prepare the onion soup mix according to package directions and pour this over the pork and potatoes.

➤ Bake at 400 degrees F (200 degrees C) for 30 to 40 minutes, or until potatoes are tender and the internal temperature of the pork reaches 160 degrees F (70 degrees C).

Pork Chops with Apples, Onions, and Sweet

Ingredients

- 4 pork chops
- salt and pepper to taste
- 2 onions, sliced into rings
- 2 sweet potatoes, sliced
- 2 apples - peeled, cored, and sliced into rings
- 3 tablespoons brown sugar
- 2 teaspoons freshly ground black pepper
- 1 teaspoon salt

Directions

- Preheat oven to 375 degrees F (190 degrees C). Season pork chops with salt and pepper to taste, and arrange in a medium oven safe skillet.

- Top pork chops with onions, sweet potatoes, and apples. Sprinkle with brown sugar. Season with 2 teaspoons pepper and 1 teaspoon salt.

- Cover, and bake 1 hour in the preheated oven, until sweet potatoes are tender and pork chops have reached an internal temperature of 160 degrees F (70 degrees C).

Indiana Potato Salad

Ingredients

- 8 baking potatoes, peeled and cubed
- 1 cup mayonnaise
- 8 ounces processed cheese food, cubed
- 1 cup chopped onion
- 8 ounces sliced bacon

Directions

- Preheat the oven to 350 degrees F (175 degrees C). Place potatoes into a pot and fill with enough water to cover. Bring to a boil and cook until easily pierced with a fork, about 12 minutes. Drain and pour into a 9x13 inch baking dish. Mix with mayonnaise, processed cheese and onion.

- While the potatoes are boiling, fry the bacon in a large skillet over medium heat until crisp. Drain and break into large pieces. Place on top of the potatoes. Bake for 1 hour in the preheated oven, until cheese is browned.

Heavenly Sweet Potatoes

Ingredients

* Vegetable cooking spray
* 1 (40 ounce) can cut sweet potato in heavy syrup, drained
* 1/4 teaspoon ground cinnamon
* 1/8 teaspoon ground ginger
* 3/4 cup SwansonB® Chicken Broth (Regular, Natural
* GoodnessB„ў or Certified Organic)
* 2 cups miniature marshmallows

Directions

➢ Spray a 1 1/2-quart casserole with cooking spray. Put the potatoes, cinnamon and ginger in an electric mixer bowl. Beat at medium speed until almost smooth.

➢ Add the broth and beat until potatoes are fluffy. Spoon the potato mixture in the prepared dish. Top with the marshmallows.

➢ Bake at 350 degrees F for 20 minutes or until heated through and marshmallows are golden brown.

Dill Potato Salad

Ingredients

- 7 cups chopped new potatoes
- 1 (8 ounce) container sour cream
- 2 teaspoons chopped fresh dill weed
- 1 teaspoon dried parsley
- 2 tablespoons Dijon mustard
- 1/2 teaspoon salt
- 1/4 teaspoon pepper

Directions

> Bring a large pot of salted water to a boil. Add potatoes and cook until tender but still firm, about 15 minutes. Drain, cool, peel and chill.

> Meanwhile, in a medium bowl combine sour cream, dill, parsley, Dijon, salt and pepper.Pour dressing over potatoes and toss gently. Chill before serving.

Red Potato Salad

Ingredients

- 3 pounds red potatoes, cut into chunks
- 1 cup low-fat sour cream
- 1/2 cup light mayonnaise
- 2 teaspoons Dijon mustard
- 1 teaspoon white vinegar
- 4 hard-cooked eggs, chopped
- 1 dill pickle, chopped
- 1/3 celery stalk, chopped
- 2 green onions, chopped
- 1 dash hot sauce
- 1 tablespoon dried dill weed
- 1/2 teaspoon garlic powder
- 1 dash onion salt
- salt and pepper to taste

Directions

➤ Place the potatoes in a pot with enough water tocover. Bring to a boil, and cook for about 10 minutes, or until easily pierced with a fork. Drain, and transfer to a large bowl to cool.

➤ In a medium bowl, mix the sour cream, mayonnaise, mustard, vinegar, eggs, pickle, celery, green onions, and hot sauce. Season with dill, garlic powder, onion salt, salt, and pepper.

➤ Pour over the potatoes, and gently toss to coat. Chill at least 3 hours in the refrigerator before serving.

Spiced Sweet Potatoes

Ingredients

- 1 1/2 cups Smucker's® Apricot Preserves
- 1/2 cup water
- 2 teaspoons lemon juice
- 1/2 teaspoon salt
- 1/2 teaspoon ground nutmeg
- 1/4 teaspoon ground cinnamon
- 4 large sweet potatoes, peeled and cut lengthwise into eight wedges

Directions

➢ Preheat oven to 400 degrees. In a heavy saucepan, combine SMUCK-ER'S® preserves and water. Over medium high heat, bring mixture to a boil; reduce heat and simmer for 5 minutes, stirring constantly.

➢ Remove mixture from heat and stir in lemon juice, salt, nutmeg and cinnamon.Arrange sweet potatoes in a baking pan. Using a pastry brush, baste potatoe thoroughly with sauce, using about half the sauce.

➢ Bake about 40 minutes, or until tender, basting with remaining sauce about halfway through cooking time.

Potato Casserole II

Ingredients

- ❀ 1/2 cup chopped onion
- ❀ 1 pint sour cream
- ❀ 1 (10.75 ounce) can condensed cream of chicken soup
- ❀ 2 cups shredded Cheddar cheese salt and pepper to taste
- ❀ 1 (2 pound) package frozen hash brown potatoes, thawed
- ❀ 2 cups crushed potato chips
- ❀ 1/2 cup melted butter

Directions

➢ Preheat oven to 350 degrees F (175 degrees C).In a large mixing bowl combine onion, sour cream, soup, cheese, salt and pepper.

➢ Press the excess water out of the hash browns and then add them to the soup mixture and mix well.

➢ Transfer to a 9x12 inch casserole dish. Sprinkle potato chips on top, then drizzle with butter.Bake in preheated oven for 45 minutes to 1 hour, until golden brown.

Ima's Potato Salad

Ingredients

- 2 pounds russet potatoes, peeled
- 3/4 cup mayonnaise
- 1 cup frozen peas and carrots, thawed
- 6 hard-cooked eggs, chopped
- 6 Israeli-style pickles, chopped
- 1/2 cup spicy mustard
- salt and pepper to taste

Directions

- Place the potatoes into a large pot and cover with salted water. Bring to a boil over high heat, then reduce heat to medium-low, cover, and simmer until tender, about 20 minutes.

- Drain and allow to steam dry for a minute or two.Finely chop the hard-cooked eggs and the pickles. When they're cool enough to handle, cube the potatoes and transfer them to a 9x13-inch dish.

- Stir in the chopped eggs, pickles, mayonnaise, mustard, and the peas and carrots and mix gently to combine. Season to taste with salt and pepper. Serve immediately, or refrigerate the salad before serving.

Meat and Potatoes Lumpia

Ingredients

- ❀ 5 medium potatoes, peeled and cut into 1/2-inch chunks
- ❀ 1 pound lean ground beef
- ❀ 1/4 cup minced onion
- ❀ 1/4 cup minced green bell pepper
- ❀ salt to taste
  ground black pepper to taste
- ❀ 1 cup frozen mixed peas and carrots, thawed
- ❀ 1 cup canola oil
- ❀ 1 (16 ounce) package egg roll wrappers

Directions

- ➢ Place potatoes in a pot with enough lightly salted water to cover, and bring to a boil. Cook 10 minutes, or until tender; drain.Place the beef, onion, and green bell pepper in a skillet over medium heat.

- ➢ Season with salt and black pepper. Cook until beef is evenly brown and onion is tender. Mix in peas and carrots, and continue cooking until heated through.

- ➢ In a large bowl, mix the potatoes with the beef mixture. Cover and refrigerate (or place in the freezer) until cooled completely.

- ➢ Heat the oil in a large skillet or deep fryer to 365 degrees F (185 degrees C). Lay egg roll wrappers on a flat surface, and place about 1/4 cup filling in the center of each.

- ➢ Fold to form egg rolls, and seal with moistened fingers.In batches, fry the egg rolls in the heated oil about 3 minutes on each side, until golden brown. Drain on paper towels.

Pleasing Cheese Potatoes

Ingredients

- 1 (32 ounce) package tater tots
- 3 eggs, lightly beaten
- 2 (10.75 ounce) cans condensed cream of potato soup, undiluted
- 1 cup sour cream
- 1/4 cup chopped green pepper
- 1/4 cup chopped onion
- 4 cups shredded Cheddar cheese

Directions

➤ Arrange Tater Tots in a greased 13-in. x 9-in. x 2-in. baking dish. In a bowl, combine the eggs, soup, sour cream, green pepper and onion until blended.

➤ Stir in the cheese. Pour over Tater tots. Bake, uncovered, at 350 degrees F for 50-55 minutes or until bubbly and golden brown. Let stand for 10 minutes before serving.

Greek Style Potatoes

Ingredients

- 1/3 cup olive oil
- 1 1/2 cups water
- 2 cloves garlic, finely chopped
- 1/4 cup fresh lemon juice
- 1 teaspoon dried thyme
- 1 teaspoon dried rosemary
- 2 cubes chicken bouillon
  ground black pepper to taste
- 6 potatoes, peeled and quartered

Directions

➤ Preheat oven to 350 degrees F (175 degrees C). In a small bowl, mix olive oil, water, garlic, lemon juice, thyme, rosemary, bouillon cubes and pepper.

➤ Arrange potatoes evenly in the bottom of a medium baking dish. Pour the olive oil mixture over the potatoes. Cover, and bake 1 1/2 to 2 hours in the preheated oven, turning occasionally, until tender but firm.

Sausage Scalloped Potatoes

Ingredients

- ❀ 1 pound fully cooked kielbasa or
- ❀ Polish sausage, cut into 1/4-inch slices
- ❀ 2 tablespoons butter or margarine
- ❀ 2 tablespoons all-purpose flour
- ❀ 1 teaspoon salt
- ❀ 1/4 teaspoon pepper
- ❀ 2 cups milk
- ❀ 4 medium red potatoes, halved and thinly sliced
- ❀ 1/4 cup chopped onion
- ❀ 2 tablespoons minced fresh parsley

Directions

➤ Place sausage in a microwave-safe bowl. Micro-wave, uncovered, on high for 3 minutes. Drain and set aside. Place butter in a 2-1/2-qt. microwave-safe dish. Heat on high for 45-60 seconds or until melted.

➤ Whisk in flour, salt and pepper until smooth. Gradually whisk in milk. Microwave, uncovered, on high for 8-10 minutes or until thickened and bubbly, stirring every 2 minutes.

➤ Stir in potatoes and onion. Cover and microwave on high for 4 minutes; stir. Heat 4 minutes longer. Stir in the sausage.

➤ Cover and cook for 8-10 minutes, stirring every 4 minutes or until potatoes are tender and sausage is heated through. Stir. Let stand, covered, for 5 minutes. Sprinkle with parsley if desired.

Red Potatoes with Beans

Ingredients

- 1 1/3 pounds fresh green beans, trimmed
- 1/3 cup water
- 6 small red potatoes, cut into wedges
- 1/2 cup chopped red onion
- 1/2 cup Italian salad dressing

Directions

➢ Place the beans and water in a 2-qt. microwave-safe dish. Cover and microwave on high for 6-8 minutes or until tender.

➢ Meanwhile, place the potatoes in a large saucepan and cover with water. Bring to a boil. Reduce heat; cover and cook for 5-7 minutes or until tender.

➢ Drain beans and potatoes; place in a bowl. Add onion and dressing; toss to coat.

Red and Sweet Potato Salad

Ingredients

- ❀ 2 pounds red potatoes, cut into 1-inch chunks
- ❀ 1 pound sweet potatoes, peeled and cut in 1-inch chunks
- ❀ 1/4 cup red wine vinegar
- ❀ 1 tablespoon spicy brown mustard
- ❀ 1 1/4 teaspoons salt
- ❀ 1/2 teaspoon pepper
- ❀ 1/2 cup reduced-fat mayonnaise
- ❀ 1/4 cup 2% milk
- ❀ 2 celery ribs, chopped
- ❀ 1 small red onion, chopped
- ❀ 1/3 cup minced fresh parsley

Directions

➢ Place the red potatoes in a large saucepan and cover with water; bring to a boil. Reduce heat; cover and cook for 2 minutes.

➢ Ad sweet potatoes; return to a boil. Reduce heat; cover and cook 8-10 minutes longer or until potatoes are fork-tender.

➢ In a large bowl, whisk the vinegar, mustard, salt and pepper. Drain potatoes; add to vinegar mixture and stir gently to coat. Cool.

➢ In a small bowl, combine mayonnaise and milk. Stir in the celery, onion and parsley. Gently stir into cooled potato mixture. Serve immediately or cover and chill.

Apple Mashed Potatoes

Ingredients

- ⚜ 4 medium potatoes, peeled and cubed
- ⚜ 2 medium tart apples, peeled and quartered
- ⚜ 1/2 teaspoon salt
- ⚜ 4 bacon strips, diced
- ⚜ 1 small onion, quartered and thinly sliced
- ⚜ 1/4 cup butter, softened
- ⚜ 1 teaspoon cider vinegar
- ⚜ 1/2 teaspoon sugar
- ⚜ 1 dash ground nutmeg

Directions

➢ Place the potatoes, apples and salt in a large saucepan; add enough water to cover. Bring to a boil; cover and cook for 12 minutes or until tender.

➢ Meanwhile, in a small skillet, cook bacon over medium heat until crisp. Remove to paper towels; drain, reserving 1 teaspoon dripp-ings. In the drippings, saute onion until tender.

➢ Drain the potatoes and apples. Add the butter, vinegar and sugar; mash until smooth. Top with bacon, onion and nutmeg.

Pimiento Potato Salad

Ingredients

- 1/2 cup mayonnaise
- 1/4 cup chopped celery
- 2 tablespoons chopped onion
- 2 tablespoons chopped pimientos
- 1 tablespoon cider vinegar
- 2 teaspoons spicy brown mustard
- 1/2 teaspoon salt
- 1/4 teaspoon pepper
- 2 cups cubed cooked potatoes
- 2 tablespoons crumbled cooked bacon

Directions

> In a bowl, whisk the mayonnaise, celery, onion, pimientos, vinegar, mustard, salt and pepper until smooth. Add potatoes and bacon; stir to coat. Refrigerate until serving.

Creamy Mashed Potatoes II

Ingredients

- ❀ 8large potatoes, peeled and cubed
- ❀ 4 ounces cream cheese
- ❀ 1/3 cup butter
- ❀ 8 ounces sour cream
- ❀ 1/2 (1 ounce) package dry Ranch-style dressing mix

Directions

➢ Preheat the oven to 350 degrees F (175 degrees C).Place potatoes in a large pot with enough water to cover.

➢ Bring to a boil, and cook until potatoes are tender, about 10 minutes. Drain water, and add cream cheese, butter, sour cream and ranch dressing mix.

➢ Mash until creamy using a potato masher or electric mixer. Spread evenly in a large baking dish.Bake for 30 minutes in the preheated oven, until the top is golden brown.

Onion Roasted Sweet Potatoes

Ingredients

- ❀ 2 (1 ounce) packages dry onion soup mix
- ❀ 2 pounds sweet potatoes, peeled and diced
- ❀ 1/3 cup vegetable oil

Directions

- ➤ Preheat oven to 450 degrees F (230 degrees C). In a large bowl, toss the dry onion soup mix, sweet potatoes and vegetable oil until the sweet potatoes are well coated.

- ➤ Arrange the mixture on a large baking sheet. Bake in the preheated oven 40 to 50 minutes, or until the sweet potatoes are tender.

Roasted Fan-Shaped Potatoes

Ingredients

* 12 large baking potatoes
* 1/2 teaspoon salt
* 1/2 cup butter or margarine, melted
* 6 tablespoons dry bread crumbs
* 6 tablespoons shredded
* Parmesan cheese

Directions

➢ With a sharp knife, slice potatoes thinly but not all the way through, leaving slices attached at the bottom. Place potatoes in a greased shallow baking dish. Sprinkle with salt; brush with 1/4 cup butter. Bake, uncovered, at 425 degrees F for 30 minutes.

➢ Brush potatoes with remaining butter and sprin-kle with bread crumbs. Bake 20 minutes longer. Sprinkle with Parmesan cheese. Bake 5-10 minutes more or until potatoes are tender and golden brown.

Sweet Potato Biscuits

Ingredients

- 2 1/2 cups all-purpose flour
- 1 tablespoon baking powder
- 1 teaspoon salt
- 1/3 cup shortening
- 1 (15 ounce) can sweet potatoes, drained
- 3/4 cup milk

Directions

- In a bowl, combine the flour, baking powder and salt. Cut in shortening until mixture resembles coarse crumbs. In another bowl, mash the sweet potatoes and milk.

- Add to the crumb mixture just until combined. Turn onto a floured surface; knead 8-10 times. Roll to 1/2-in. thickness; cut with a 2-1/2-in.

- biscuit cutter. Place on ungreased baking sheets. Bake at 425 degrees F for 8-10 minutes or until golden brown. Remove to wire racks. Serve warm.

Butterscotch Potato Chip Cookies

Ingredients

- 1 cup packed brown sugar
- 1 cup white sugar
- 1 cup butter
- 2 eggs
- 2 1/2 cups all-purpose flour
- 1 teaspoon baking soda
- 1 1/3 cups butterscotch chips
- 2 cups crushed potato chips

Directions

➢ Preheat oven to 350 degrees F (180 degrees C). Cream together sugars and butter or margarine. Beat in eggs, add flour and baking soda, mix well.

➢ Fold in butterscotch chips and potato chips. Drop by tsp. on cookie sheet and bake for 8 to 10 minutes.

Sweet Potato Pie

Ingredients

- 2 pounds sweet potatoes
- 3/4 cup packed brown sugar
- 1/4 cup all-purpose flour
- 2 teaspoons grated orange peel
- 1 teaspoon pumpkin pie spice
- 1 teaspoon vanilla extract
- 1/8 teaspoon salt
- 1 cup fat-free milk
- 1/2 cup egg substitute
- 1 (9 inch) unbaked pastry shell
- 1/2 cup reduced-fat whipped topping

Directions

- Bake sweet potatoes at 350 degrees F for 1 hour or until very soft. Cool slightly. Cut potatoes in half; scoop out the pulp and discard shells. Place pulp in a food processor or blender; cover and process until smooth.

- In a bowl, combine the pulp, brown sugar, flour, orange peel, pumpkin pie spice, vanilla and salt. Stir in milk and egg substitute until we blended. Pour into pastry shell.

- Bake at 375 degrees F for 45-50 minutes or until a knife inserted near the center comes out clean. Cool on a wire rack for 2 hours. Garnish with whipped topping. Refrigerate leftovers.

Oven-Crisped Potatoes

Ingredients

- 2 medium potatoes, peeled and thinly sliced
- 3 tablespoons butter or margarine, melted
- 1 tablespoon finely chopped onion
- 1/8 teaspoon pepper

Directions

➢ Arrange potatoes in an ungreased 1-1/2-qt. baking dish. Combine butter, onion and pepper; pour over potatoes. Bake, uncovered, at 425 degrees F for 1 hour or until potatoes are tender.

Baked Potato Dip

Ingredients

- 2 (16 ounce) containers sour cream
- 1 (3 ounce) can bacon bits
- 2 cups shredded Cheddar cheese
- 1 bunch green onions, chopped

Directions

➢ In a medium size mixing bowl, combine sour cream, bacon, Cheddar cheese and green onions; stir well. Refrigerate, or serve immediately.

Spicy Pumpkin and Sweet Potato Soup

Ingredients

* 1 tablespoon coriander seeds
* 2 teaspoons cumin seeds
* 2 teaspoons dried oregano
* 1 tablespoon fennel seeds
* 1/2 teaspoon crushed red pepper
* 1/2 teaspoon salt
* 1/2 teaspoon whole black peppercorns
* 1 clove garlic
* 2 tablespoons olive oil, divided
* 1 medium sugar pumpkin
* 4 orange-fleshed sweet potatoes
* 1 large onion, chopped
* 1 1/2 quarts chicken broth

Direction

➤ Preheat oven to 400 degrees F (200 degrees C). In a mortar or spice grinder, grind coriander, cumin, oregano, fennel, red pepper, salt and peppercorns into a coarse powder. Blend in garlic and 1 tablespoon olive oil to form a paste.

➤ Wash pumpkin, and cut into 2-inch wide wedges, scraping away seeds. Peel potatoes and cut each potato lengthwise into 6 wedges.

➤ Smear the pumpkin and the potatoes with the spice paste and place in a baking dish.Roast in preheated oven 30 to 40 minutes, until tender and just beginning to blacken at the thinnest points.

➤ Meanwhile, in a large pot over medium heat, cook the onion in the remaining 1 tablespoon olive oil until translucent.Chop pumpkin and potatoes into smaller chunks and puree in a blender or food processor with some of the chicken broth until smooth.

➤ Be sure to scrape the roasted spice paste off the baking dish and include it in the puree. It may be necessary to deglaze the dish with a little chicken broth.

➤ Pour the pureed vegetables into the pot with the onions, and stir in as much additional chicken stock as needed to achieve the desired consistency. Heat through.

Jeannie's Famous Potato Hamburger Casserolex

Ingredients

- ❀ 1 tablespoon olive oil
- ❀ 1 yellow onion, thinly sliced
- ❀ 1 pound ground beef
- ❀ 1/4 cup butter
- ❀ 1/4 cup all-purpose flour
- ❀ 3 cups milk
- ❀ 1 pint heavy cream
- ❀ salt and pepper to taste
- ❀ 5 potatoes, sliced
- ❀ 2 cups shredded Cheddar cheese
- ❀ 2 cups shredded Monterey Jack cheese
- ❀ 1 cup milk

Directions

➢ Preheat oven to 350 degrees F (175 degrees C).Heat oil in a large heavy skillet over medium heat. Cook and stir onions until translucent; set aside.

➢ Cook ground beef until evenly brown. Drain excess fat, and set beef aside. Melt butter in the skillet. Add flour, and stir with a whisk for 5 minutes. Gradually whisk in 3 cups milk, then the cream.

➢ Simmer, stirringfrequently, over medium-low heat for 10 minutes until the sauce has thickened and is smooth. Season with salt and pepper, and remove from heat.

➢ Spread a small amount of sauce in the bottom of a 9x13 inch casserole dish. Alternate layers of potatoes, onions, ground beef, cheese and sauce, with 2 to 3 layers of each. Reserve some cheese to sprinkle on top.

➢ If you run short of sauce, press down on all layers, and add milk as needed. Sprinkle remaining cheese on top.Bake in preheated oven for 45 to 55 minutes, or until potatoes are soft.

Dar's Super Savory Sauerkraut Potato Bake

Ingredients

- 1/3 cup all-purpose flour
- 2 teaspoons chicken bouillon granules
- 1 cup water
- 1 cup milk
- 1/4 cup sour cream
- 1 small onion, finely chopped
- 1 cup shredded Cheddar cheese
- 1 cup drained sauerkraut
- 1/2 teaspoon salt
- 1/2 teaspoon ground black pepper
- 1/2 teaspoon caraway seeds (optional)
- 3 tablespoons unsalted butter, melted
- 1 (16 ounce) package frozen
- shredded hash brown potatoes

Directions

- Preheat an oven to 350 degrees F (175 degrees C). Grease a 9x13-inch baking dish.Whisk the flour, bouillon granules, water, and milk together in a medium saucepan; bring to a boil until thick, 1 to 2 minutes, whisking continuously.

- Remove from heat and stir the sour cream into the flour mixture; set aside to cool.Combine the onion, Cheddar cheese,sauerkraut, salt, pepper, and caraway seeds in a large mixing bowl.

- Stir the sour cream sauce and the melted butter into the sauerkraut mixture; fold the hashb brown potatoes into the mixture.

- Pour into the prepared baking dish. Use a spatula to flatten into an even layer.Bake in the preheated oven until the potatoes are tender and the top is brown and bubbly, 60 to 70 minutes.

Mom's Red Scalloped Potatoes

Ingredients

- 8 large red potatoes
- 3 tablespoons butter
- 1 onion, chopped
- 2 cloves garlic, chopped
- 1 (10.75 ounce) can condensed cream of broccoli soup
- 1 (10.75 ounce) can condensed cream of celery soup
- 1 cup milk
- salt and pepper to taste
- 4 cups shredded Cheddar cheese

Directions

- Preheat an oven to 350 degrees F (175 degrees C). Butter a large baking dish. Wash and peel the potatoes so that only some of the peel remains on the potatoes; cut into 1/8 inch slices.

- Put the potatoes in the prepared dish.Melt the butter in a large pot over medium-high heat

- Cook the onion and garlic in the melted butter until soft and translucent, 7 to 10 minutes; stir in the broccoli soup, celery soup, milk, salt, pepper, and about half of the Cheddar cheese; cook until the cheese has melted.

- Pour the mixture over the potatoes; top with the remaining Cheddar cheese. Cover with aluminum foil or lid.

- Bake in the preheated oven for 45 minutes. Remove the cover and cook until the cheese begins to brown, about 10 minutes more.

Harvest Sweet Potato Pie

Ingredients

- 4 eggs
- 1 (12 ounce) can evaporated milk
- 1 1/4 cups sugar
- 3/4 cup butter or margarine, melted
- 2 teaspoons ground cinnamon
- 2 teaspoons pumpkin pie spice
- 1 teaspoon vanilla extract
- 1 teaspoon lemon extract
- 1/2 teaspoon ground nutmeg
- 1/2 teaspoon salt
- 4 cups mashed cooked sweet potatoes
- 2 (9 inch) unbaked pastry shells Whipped cream

Directions

- In a mixing bowl, combine first 10 ingredients; mix well. Beat in sweet potatoes. Pour into pie shells.

- Bake at 425 degrees F for 15 minutes. Reduce heat to 350 degrees F; bake 30-35 minutes longer or until a knife inserted near the center comes out clean. Cool completely. Serve with whipped cream if desired. Store in the refrigerator.

Sweet Potato Mini Loaves

Ingredients

- 4 eggs
- 2 cups sugar
- 2 cups cold mashed sweet potatoes
- 3/4 cup vegetable oil
- 2 cups all-purpose flour
- 1 1/2 cups whole wheat flour
- 1 1/2 teaspoons ground cinnamon
- 1 teaspoon baking soda
- 1 teaspoon ground nutmeg
- 1/2 teaspoon salt
- 2/3 cup water

Directions

➢ In a large mixing bowl, beat the eggs, sugar, sweet potatoes and oil. Combine the flours, cinnamon, baking soda, nutmeg and salt; add to sweet potato mixture alternately with water.

➢ Pour into six greased 5-3/4-in. x 3-in. x 2-in. loaf pans. Bake at 350 degrees F for 30-35 minutes or until a toothpick inserted near the center comes out clean. Cool for 10 minutes before removing from pans to wire racks.

Dylan's Potato, Carrot, and Cheddar Soup

Ingredients

- 2 tablespoons olive oil
- 6 yellow potatoes, cubed
- 3 large carrots, peeled and diced
- 1 pinch salt, to taste
- 1 teaspoon garlic powder
- 1 teaspoon onion powder
- 1 (32 ounce) carton chicken broth (such as Swanson®)
- 3/4 cup shredded sharp Cheddar cheese
- 1/4 cup chopped fresh flat-leaf parsley

Directions

➤ Heat the olive oil in a pot over medium heat; cook and stir the potatoes and carrots in the hot oil until hot, about 10 minutes.

➤ Season with salt, garlic powder, and onion powder. Pour the chicken broth over the mixture; continue cooking until the potatoes and carrots are soft, 10 to 15 minutes more.

➤ Pour about half of the potato-and-carrot mixture into a blender. Hold the lid of the blender with a folded kitchen towel and carefully start the blender, using a few quick pulses to get the soup moving before leaving it on to puree.

➤ Return the pureed soup to the pot. Stir the Cheddar cheese into the soup until melted. Ladle the soup into bowls and garnish with parsley to serve.

Baked Mashed Potatoes

Ingredients

- 5 pounds Yukon Gold potatoes, peeled and cubed
- 1/2 cup butter
- 1/4 cup milk
- 1 (8 ounce) package cream cheese, softened
- 1 onion, grated
- 1 egg
- salt and pepper to taste

Directions

➤ Preheat oven to 350 degrees F (175 degrees C).Bring a large pot of lightly salted water to a boil. Add potatoes, and cook until tender but firm, about 15 minutes; drain.

➤ In a large bowl, mash potatoes with the butter and milk. With a hand mixer, beat in cream cheese and onion. In a small bowl, beat the egg with a little bit of the mashed potatoes.

➤ Stir into potatoes, and season with salt and pepper.Transfer to a 2 quart casserole dish.Bake 1 hour in the preheated oven, or until puffy and lightly browned.

Light 'n' Creamy Mashed Potatoes

Ingredients

- 3 pounds potatoes, peeled and quartered
- 4 ounces fat-free cream cheese, cubed
- 1/2 cup reduced-fat sour cream
- 1/2 cup fat-free milk
- 3/4 teaspoon salt
- 1/4 teaspoon garlic powder
- 1/4 teaspoon pepper
- 1 tablespoon minced chives
- 1 dash paprika

Directions

➢ Place potatoes in a saucepan and cover with water. Bring to a boil. Reduce heat; cover and cook for 10-15 minutes or until tender.

➢ Drain .In a large mixing bowl, mash the potatoes. Add the cream cheese, sour cream, milk, salt, garlic powder and pepper; beat until smooth. Stir in chives. Sprinkle with paprika.

Scalloped Potatoes and Hamburger

Ingredients

- 1 pound ground beef
- 6 medium potatoes, peeled and sliced
- 1 large onion, sliced
- salt and pepper to taste
- 1 (10.75 ounce) can condensed cream of mushroom soup,
- undiluted
- 1 cup milk
- 1/4 cup chopped green pepper

Directions

➢ In a skillet, cook beef over medium heat until no longer pink; drain. In a greased 13-in. x 9-in. x 2-in. baking dish, layer half of the potatoes, onion and beef; sprinkle with salt and pepper.

➢ Repeat layers. In a bowl, combine the soup, milk and green pepper; mix well. Pour over top. Cover and bake at 350 degrees F for 45 minutes. Uncover; bake 15 minutes longer or until potatoes are tender.

Salsa Chicken and Potato Packets

Ingredients

- 4 skinless, boneless chicken breast halves
- 2 cups salsa
- 4 potatoes, peeled

Directions

➢ Preheat oven to 350 degrees F (175 degrees C).Place each chicken breast in the middle of a square piece of foil. Pour 1/4 cup salsa over each breast.

➢ Slice the potatoes thin and place potato slices on top of chicken and salsa. Spoon another 1/4 cup salsa over each chicken/ potato combination.

➢ Fold foil up to form 'packets'. Place packets seam side up on a cookie sheet and bake in the preheated oven for 45 minutes. Open packets and serve.

German Potato Salad

Ingredients

- 6 bacon strips, diced
- 7 medium unpeeled red potatoes, cubed
- 2 medium onions, thinly sliced
- 1/3 cup cider vinegar
- 1/3 cup water
- 2 tablespoons sugar
- 3 tablespoons minced fresh parsley, divided
- 1 teaspoon salt
- 1 teaspoon prepared mustard
- 1/4 teaspoon pepper

Directions

- In a pressure cooker, cook bacon over medium heat until crisp; drain. Add potatoes and onions. In a bowl, combine the vinegar, water, sugar, 2 tablespoons of parsley, salt, mustard and pepper; pour over potatoes.

- Close cover securely; place pressure regulator on vent pipe. Bring cooker to full pressure over high heat. Reduce heat to medium and cook for 5 minutes.

- (Pressure regulator should maintain a slow steady rocking motion or release of steam; adjust heat if needed.)

- Remove from the heat. Immediately cool according to manufac-turer's directions until pressure is completely reduced. Just before serving, sprinkle with remaining parsley.

Potato-Topped Chili Loaf

Ingredients

- 3/4 cup diced onion
- 1/3 cup saltine crumbs
- 1 egg
- 3 tablespoons milk
- 1 tablespoon chili powder
- 1/2 teaspoon salt
- 1 1/2 pounds ground beef TOPPING:
- 3 cups hot mashed potatoes
  (prepared with milk and butter)
- 1 (11 ounce) can Mexicorn, drained
- 1 (15.5 ounce) can kidney beans, rinsed and drained
- 1/4 cup thinly sliced green onions
- 1 cup shredded Cheddar or taco cheese, divided

Directions

➤ Combine the first six ingredients; crumble beef over mixture and mix well. Press into an ungreased 9-in. square baking pan. Bake at 375 degrees F for 25 minutes or until no longer pink; drain.

➤ Combine the potatoes, corn, beans, onions and 1/2 cup of cheese; spread over meat loaf. Sprinkle with the remaining cheese. Bake 15 minutes longer or until the potato layer is lightly browned and heated through.

Sour Cream and Chive Mashed Potatoes

Ingredients

- 2 pounds Yukon Gold potatoes, peeled and quartered
- 1/2 cup milk
- 1/2 cup sour cream
- 1/4 cup chopped fresh chives
- salt and pepper to taste

Directions

➤ Place potatoes in a large pot with enough water to come up 2 inches from the bottom. Bring to a boil, and cook for 20 to 25 minutes, until fork tender.

➤ Drain, and mash. Mix in the milk using a potato masher or an electric mixer until fluffy. Stir in the sour cream and chives, and season with salt and pepper

➤

Potato Chip Cookies VII

Ingredients

- 1/2 cup butter, softened
- 1/4 cup brown sugar
- 1/4 cup white sugar
- 1/2cup applesauce
- 1 3/4 cups all-purpose flour 1/3 cup rolled oats
- 3/4 cup chopped almonds
- 3/4 cup crushed plain potato chips

Directions

➤ Preheat oven to 350 degrees F (175 degrees C). Grease cookie sheets.In a medium bowl, cream together the butter, brown sugar and white sugar until smooth.

➤ Mix in applesauce. Stir in the flour and oats, then mix in the almonds and potato chips. Drop by rounded spoonfuls onto the prepared cookie sheets.

➤ Bake for 10 to 15 minutes in the preheated oven. Allow cookies to cool on baking sheet for 5 minutes before removing to a wire rack to cool completely.

Campfire Roasted Potatoes

Ingredients

- 5 large red potatoes, cubed
- 1 medium onion, sliced
- 1 clove garlic, minced 1/4 cup butter or margarine, softened
- 3/4 teaspoon ground black pepper
- 3/4 teaspoon dried oregano salt to taste
- 1/4 cup shredded Parmesan cheese (optional)

Directions

➢ Toss together the potato, onion, garlic, butter, pepper, oregano, salt, and Parmesan cheese in a large bowl, or a resealable bag. Remove from bag, and wrap in several layers of aluminum foil, sealing the edges well.

➢ Cook on a wire rack over the hot coals of a fire, flipping over midway through cooking, until the potatoes are tender; about 30 to 40 minutes.

➢ Alternatively, the potato packet may be baked on a cookie sheet in a 350 degrees F (175 degrees C) oven.

Bacon-Potato Burritos

Ingredients

- 8 bacon strips
- 1 1/2 cups frozen Southern-style hash brown potatoes
- 2 teaspoons dried minced onion
- 4 eggs
- 1/4 cup milk
- 1 teaspoon Worcestershire sauce
- 1/4 teaspoon salt
- 1/4 teaspoon pepper
- 1 cup shredded Cheddar cheese
- 6 (8 inch) (8 inch) flour tortillas

Directions

➢ In a large skillet, cook bacon until crisp;drain on paper towels. Brown potatoes and onion in drippings.

➢ In a bowl, beat eggs; add milk,c Worcestershiresauce, salt and pepper. Pour over potatoes; cook and stir until eggs are set. Crumble bacon and stir into eggs.

➢ Sprinkle with cheese. Meanwhile, warm tortillas according to package directions. Spoon egg mixture down center of tortillas; fold in sides of tortilla. Serve with salsa.

Ham Potato Scallop

Ingredients

- ❀ 1 (5.5 ounce) package scalloped potato mix
- ❀ 2 cups boiling water
- ❀ 2 tablespoons butter or margarine
- ❀ 3/4 cup milk
- ❀ 2 cups cubed fully cooked ham
- ❀ 1 (10 ounce) package frozen cut green beans
- ❀ 1 cup shredded Cheddar cheese

Directions

➢ In a ungreased 1-1/2-qt. baking dish, combine potatoes with sauce mix, boiling water and butter. Stir in milk, ham and beans.

➢ Bake,uncovered, at 400 degrees F for 35 minutes or until the potatoes are tender, stirring occasionally. Sprinkle with cheese. Bake 5 minutes longer or until cheese is melted. let stand 5 minutes before serving.

Swiss Potatoes Gratin

Ingredients

- 1 teaspoon butter
- 2 pounds red potatoes, thinly sliced
- 1 cup ricotta cheese
- 3/4 cup chopped fresh parsley salt and pepper to taste
- 2 pinches ground nutmeg
- 1 egg
- 1 cup heavy cream
- 2 cups shredded Gruyere cheese

Directions

➢ Preheat the oven to 350 degrees F (175 degrees C). Butter a 9x13 inch baking dish.Place the potatoes into a large pot of salted water. Bring to a boil, and boil for 1 minute. Drain, rinse in cold water to cool, drain again, and pat dry.

➢ In a medium bowl, stir together the ricotta cheese, parsley, salt, pepper and nutmeg. In a measuring cup, whisk the egg with a fork, then fill the cup with enough cream to make 1 cup.

➢ Season with salt, pepper and nutmeg also.Arrange a layer of slightly overlapping potato slices in the bottom of the buttered baking dish. Dot with 1/3 of the ricotta cheese.

➢ Sprinkle with 1/3 of the Gruyere cheese. Repeat layers two more times, and end with a layer of potatoes on top. Pour the egg and cream evenly over the potatoes.

➢ Bake for 35 to 45 minutes in the preheated oven, until the potatoes are tender, and the cheese is browned and bubbly. Let rest for 10 minutes before serving to allow the sauce to thicken.

Belle's Cheesy Potato Stoup

Ingredients

- 6 potatoes, diced
- 1 (10.75 ounce) can condensed cream of onion soup
- 1 (12 ounce) can fully cooked luncheon meat (such as SPAM®), cubed
- 2 cups milk
- 1 (8 ounce) package shredded Cheddar cheese
- 1 pinch red pepper flakes, or to taste
- salt and pepper to taste

Directions

- ➤ Place the potatoes into a large saucepan and cover with salted water. Bring to a boil over high heat, then reduce heat to medium-low, cover, and simmer until the potatoes are tender, 10 to 15minutes.

- ➤ Drain off all but 2 cups of the water, then stir in the cream of onion soup, luncheon meat, milk, and Cheddar cheese. Return to a simmer over medium heat, and cook a few minutes until hot.Season to taste with red pepper flakes, salt, and pepper.

Sweet Potato Casserole II

Ingredients

- 4 1/2 cups cooked and mashed sweet potatoes
- 1/2 cup butter, melted
- 1/3 cup milk
- 1 cup white sugar
- 1/2 teaspoon vanilla extract
- 2 eggs, beaten
- 1 cup light brown sugar
- 1/2 cup all-purpose flour
- 1/3 cup butter
- 1 cup chopped pecans

Directions

- Preheat oven to 350 degrees F (175 degrees C). Grease a 9x13 inch baking dish.In a large bowl, mix together mashed sweet potatoes, 1/2 cup butter, milk, sugar, vanilla extract, and eggs.

- Spread sweet potato mixture into the prepared baking dish. In a small bowl, mix together brown sugar and flour.

- Cut in 1/3 cup butter until mixture is crumbly, then stir in pecans. Sprinkle pecan mixture over the sweet potatoes.Bake for 25 minutes in the preheated oven, or until golden brown.

My Potato Pudding

Ingredients

- 6 medium potatoes, peeled
- 7 eggs
- 2 tablespoons vegetable oil
- 1 onion, grated
- 1/3 cup matzo meal
- 1 teaspoon baking powder
- 1/2 teaspoon salt, or to taste
- 1/2 teaspoon ground black pepper, or to taste
- 2 tablespoons vegetable oil

Directions

➤ Preheat the oven to 350 degrees F (175 degrees C). Generously grease two 8 inch square baking dishes.

➤ Shred the potatoes and place them in a bowl of cold water to prevent discolor-ration. In a large bowl, beat the eggs and 2 Table-spoons of oil together.

➤ Stir in the onion. Drain the potatoes, and stir them into the egg mixture as well. Gradually mix in the matzo meal and baking powder.

➤ Season with salt and pepper. Divide the mixture between the two prepared pans, and spread evenly. Drizzle or brush remaining oil over the top.Bake for 1 hour in the preheated oven, or until nicely browned. Serve hot or cold.

PHILLY Mini Potato Bites

Ingredients

- 1 1/2 pounds new potatoes
- 1/2 cup PHILADELPHIA Herb & Garlic Cream Cheese Spread
- 2 tablespoons sour cream
- 2 tablespoons KRAFT 100% Parmesan Grated Cheese
- 2 tablespoons OSCAR MAYER Real Bacon Bits
- 2 tablespoons chopped fresh chives

Directions

- Place potatoes in large saucepan; add enough water to cover. Bring to boil on medium-high heat. Reduce heat to medium-low; simmer15 minutes or until potatoes are tender.

- Meanwhile, mix cream cheese spread, sour cream and Parmesan cheese; cover. Refrigerate until ready to use.

- Drain potatoes. Cool slightly. Cut potatoes in half; cut small piece from rounded bottom of each potato half.

- Place, bottom-sidesdown, on serving platter. Top each with 1 teaspoon of the cream cheese mixture. Sprinkle evenly with bacon bits and chives.

Tasty Potato Latkes\

Ingredients

- ❋ 2 cups peeled and shredded potatoes
- ❋ 2 tablespoons dry onion soup mix
- ❋ 2 cloves garlic, minced
- ❋ 2 eggs, beaten
- ❋ 2 tablespoons all-purpose flour
- ❋ 1/3 cup shredded Cheddar
- ❋ cheese
- ❋ 1 teaspoon salt
- ❋ cracked black pepper to taste
- ❋ 1/2 cup vegetable oil
- ❋ 1tablespoon chopped green onion for garnish
- ❋ 1tablespoon sour cream for garnish

Directions

➤ Place the shredded potatoes in a cloth, and wring as much of the moisture out as possible. Place the potatoes into a bowl, and stir in the onion soup mix, garlic, eggs, flour, Cheddar cheese, salt, and pepper until well mixed.

➤ Heat the vegetable oil in a large skillet over medium heat until it shimmers, and drop the potato mixture by heaping tablespoons into the hot oil. Press down on the patties to flatten them to about 1/3 inch thick.

➤ Fry the patties until golden brown and crisp on the bottoms, 5 to 8 minutes, then flip and cook the other side until crisp and golden.

➤ Remove the latkes to paper towels to drain, and serve hot, sprinkled with green onion and a small dollop of sour cream.

Pressure Cooker Potato Salad

Ingredients

- 6 medium red potatoes, scrubbed
- 1 cup water
- 1/4 cup chopped onion
- 1stalk celery, chopped
- salt and pepper to taste
- 3 hard-cooked eggs, chopped
- 1 tablespoon chopped fresh dill
- 1/2 cup mayonnaise
- 1 teaspoon yellow mustard
- 1 teaspoon cider vinegar

Directions

➢ Place potatoes in pressure cooker with water. Cook on high pressure 3 minutes. If potatoes are larger, cook for 4 minutes.

➢ Let steam release for 3 minutes. Then quickly release pressure and open cooker. Peel and dice potatoes when they are cool enough to handle.

➢ Alternate layers of potatoes, onion, and celery in a large bowl. Season each layer with salt and pepper. Top with the chopped egg and sprinkle with dill.

➢ Mix together the mayonnaise, mustard, and cider vinegar in a small bowl. Gently fold the mayonnaise mixture into the potatoes. Chill at least one hour before serving.

Herbed Garlic Mashed Potatoes

Ingredients

- 1 medium head garlic
- 1/2 cup low fat, low sodium chicken broth
- 3 potatoes, peeled and cubed
- 1 cup warm skim milk
- 2 tablespoons olive oil
- 1 tablespoon dried thyme
- 1/2 teaspoon dried rosemary, crushed
- salt and pepper to taste

Directions

➢ Preheat oven to 350 degrees F (175 degrees C).Slice the top off the head of garlic to expose the cloves. Place the whole head and the broth in a small casserole dish and cover.

➢ Bake for 1 hour; remove dish from the oven and set aside.Boil the cubed potatoes in water for 20 minutes or until soft. Drain.

➢ Add the warm milk and olive oil. Beat with mixer until potatoes are fluffy. Add the herbs.Gently squeeze the garlic out from each of the cloves, leaving behind the skins.

➢ Add all the garlic pulp to the potatoes. Beat again and season with salt and pepper.

Sweet Potato Pie I

Ingredients

- 1 (1 pound) sweet potato
- 1/2 cup butter, softened
- 1 cup white sugar
- 1/2 cup milk
- 2 eggs
- 1/2 teaspoon ground nutmeg
- 1/2 teaspoon ground cinnamon
- 1 teaspoon vanilla extract
- 1 (9 inch) unbaked pie crust

Directions

> Boil sweet potato whole in skin for 40 to 50 minutes, or until done. Run cold water over the sweet potato, and remove the skin. Break apart sweet potato in a bowl. Add butter, and mix well with mixer.

> Stir in sugar, milk, eggs, nutmeg, cinnamon and vanilla. Beat on medium speed until mixture is smooth. Pour filling into an unbaked pie crust.

> Bake at 350 degrees F (175 degrees C) for 55 to 60 minutes, or until knife inserted in center comes out clean. Pie will puff up like a souffle, and then will sink down as it cools.

Pork Loin with Potatoes

Ingredients

* 1 (5 pound) bone-in pork loin roast
* 3 cloves garlic, sliced
* 3tablespoons olive oil
* 1/4teaspoonpaprika
* 1/4 teaspoon pepper
* 1/8 teaspoon dried thyme
* 6 medium potatoes, peele
* 1/2 teaspoon salt
* ONION MUSHROOM GRAVY:
* 1 cup water
* 1 cup beef broth
* 2 medium onions, sliced
* 1 1/4 cups chopped fresh mushrooms
* 1 tablespoon butter
* 1 tablespoon vegetable oil
* 1/4 cup all-purpose flour
* 2 tablespoons minced fresh parsley
* 1/4 teaspoon pepper

Directions

➤ Cut slits in top of roast; insert garlic slices. Combine the oil, paprika, pepper and thyme; rub over roast. Place in a large resealable plastic bag; seal and refrigerate the roast overnight.

➤ Transfer roast to a shallow roasting pan. bake, uncovered, at 350 degrees F for 1-3/4 hours.Meanwhile, place potatoes and salt in a saucepan and cover with water.

➤ Bring to boil. Reduce heat; simmer, uncovered, for 15 minutes or until almost tender. Drain; cool slightly. Cut potatoes into quarters; arrange around roast.

➤ Bake 45 minutes longer or until a meat thermo-meter reads 160 degrees F and potatoes are tender, basting potatoes with drippings occasionally.

➤ Remove potatoes; keep warm. Cover roast and let stand for 15 minutes before carving.For gravy, pourdrippings and loosened browned bits into a measuring cup.

➤ Skim fat, reserving 2 tablespoonsdrippings. Add water and broth to reserved drippings; set aside. In a large saucepan, saute onions and mushrooms in

91

butter and oil until tender.

➤ Stir in flour until blended. Gradually stir in broth mixture. Bring to a boil; cook and stir for 2 minutes or until thickened. Stir in parsley and pepper. Serve with roast and potatoes.

Mashed Potato Tacos

Ingredients

- 2 cups dry potato flakes
- 6 hard taco shells
- 2 tablespoons butter
- 1/2 cup sour cream
- 1/2 cup shredded Cheddar cheese
- 1/2 cup French-fried onions taco sauce

Directions

- Prepare the dry potato flakes according to package directions. Warm the taco shells according to package directions.

- In a bowl, mix the prepared mashed potatoes, butter, sour cream, Cheddar cheese, and French-fried onions.

- Fill the taco shells with the mashed potato mixture, and serve with taco sauce.

Scalloped Potatoes II

Ingredients

- 3 pounds potatoes, thinly sliced salt to taste
- 9 tablespoons all-purpose flour
- 6 tablespoons butter, diced
- 1 quart milk

Directions

- Preheat oven to 425 degrees F (220 degrees C). Grease a 9x13 inch baking dish.Arrange one layer of potatoes in the bottom of the prepared baking dish.

- Sprinkle the potatoes with salt, 3 tablespoons flour and 2tablespoons butter. Repeat layering 2 more times, until all of potatoes have been used.

- Slowly pour milk over the potatoes until the dish is 3/4 full of milk.Bake until the milk comes to a boil (check after 5 minutes), then reduce heat to 375 degrees F (190 degrees C) for another 45 to 60 minutes.

Zesty Potato Soup

Ingredients

- 4 large potatoes, peeled and cubed
- 2 cups water
- 1 teaspoon dried minced onion
- 1 garlic clove, minced
- 1/2 teaspoon salt
- 1/4 teaspoon pepper
- 1 cup milk
- 4 ounces process American cheese, cubed
- 1/3 cup chopped green chilies
- 2 tablespoons butter
- 1 tablespoon chicken bouillon granules
- 2 teaspoons minced fresh parsley

Directions

- In a large saucepan, combine the potatoes, water, onion, garlic, salt and pepper; bring to a boil over medium heat. Reduce heat; cover and simmer for 15-20 minutes or until potatoes are tender (Do not drain.)

- Mash potatoes in liquid until almost smooth. Add remaining ingredients; cook and stir until cheese is melted.

Potato Chicken Stew

Ingredients

- 4 cups cooked, cubed chicken breast meat
- 2/3 cup sliced fresh mushrooms
- 1 cup chopped onion, sauteed in butter
- 1 1/2 cups chopped carrots
- 6 cups chicken stock
- 1 teaspoon dried sage
- 1 teaspoon dried basil leaves
- 1 teaspoon garlic salt
- 1 teaspoon dried parsley
- 1 (10 ounce) package frozen mixed vegetables, thawed
- 3 cups cooked, diced red potatoes
- 1/2 cup chopped celery
- 1/8 cup all-purpose flour

Directions

- Combine chicken, mushrooms, onion, carrots and stock in a large saucepan over medium heat. Simmer until carrots are tender, about 10 minutes.

- Stir in sage, basil, garlic salt, parsley, mixed vegetables, potatoes and celery and cook until heated through. Stir in flour to thicken sauce, then serve.

Potato Pizza Casserole

Ingredients

- 1 pound ground beef
- 1 small onion, chopped
- salt and pepper to taste
- 1/4 teaspoon garlic powder
- 5 cups peeled and thinly sliced potatoes
- 1 (3 ounce) package chopped pepperoni
- 1 (10.75 ounce) can condensed tomato soup
- 1 (10.75 ounce) can condensed Cheddar cheese soup
- 1/2 cup milk
- 1/2 teaspoon dried oregano
- 1/4 teaspoon Italian seasoning
- 1/2 teaspoon brown sugar
- 8 ounces shredded mozzarella cheese

Directions

- Preheat the oven to 350 degrees F (175 degrees C). Cook the ground beef and onion in a large skillet over medium heat until evenly browned.

- Drain off grease. Season with salt, pepper, and garlic powder.Spread the sliced potatoes in a layer on the bottom of a 9x13 inch baking dish.

- Spread the ground beef and onion over the potatoes. Place slices of pepperoni over the ground beef. In a saucepan over medium heat, combine the tomato soup, Cheddar cheese soup,and milk.

- Season with oregano, Ital ian seasoning, and brown sugar. Mix well, and cook until heated through. Pour over the contents of the baking dish.

- Cover the dish with aluminum foil, and bake for 30 minutes in the preheated oven. Remove the aluminum foil, sprinkle mozzarella cheese over the top, and bake for an additional 15 minutes, until the cheese is melted and bubbly.

New Potatoes with Caper Sauce

Ingredients

- 12 small new potatoes, scrubbed
- 1/2 cup butter, softened
- 2 tablespoons capers, chopped
- 1 tablespoon minced green onion
- 1/3 cup grated Parmesan cheese
- 2 tablespoons chopped fresh parsley
- 1 teaspoon white wine vinegar
- salt and pepper to taste

Directions

- ➤ Combine the softened butter, capers, green onion, Parmesan cheese, parsley and vinegar in a bowl. Set aside.

- ➤ Bring a large pot of salted water to a boil. If potatoes are large, cut into halves or quarters. Add potatoes and cook until tender but still firm, 15 to 20 minutes. Drain.

- ➤ Add the caper sauce to the pot of drained potatoes and toss gently to coat. Season to taste with salt and pepper.

Sweet Potato Pie

Ingredients

- ❀ 1 1/2 cups sugar
- ❀ 2 teaspoons all-purpose flour
- ❀ 1 (5 ounce) can evaporated milk
- ❀ 1 egg, lightly beaten
- ❀ 1 teaspoon vanilla extract
- ❀ 2 cups mashed cooked sweet potatoes
- ❀ 1 (9 inch) unbaked pastry shell GLAZE:
- ❀ 1/2 cup sugar
- ❀ 2 1/4 teaspoons all-purpose flour
- ❀ 2 tablespoons butter or margarine, melted
- ❀ 2tablespoons evaporated milk
- ❀ 1/4 cup pecan halves

Directions

➢ In a bowl, combine sugar, flour, milk, egg and vanilla. Stir in the sweet potatoes. Pour into pastry shell.

➢ For glaze, combine the sugar, flour, butter and milk; drizzle over sweet potato mixture. Garnish with pecans. Cover edges of pastry loosely with foil.

➢ Bake at 375 degrees for 45 minutes. Remove foil; bake 15 minutes longer or until crust is golden brown and a knife inserted near the center comes out clean.

Marinated Potato Salad with Anchovy Vinaigrette

Ingredients

- 1 1/2 cups vegetable oil
- 1/2 cup white wine vinegar
- 1/4 cup chopped parsley
- 1 1/2 teaspoons salt
- 1 teaspoon white sugar
- 1 (2 ounce) can anchovy filets
- 2 cloves garlic, minced
- 3 pounds red potatoes
- 1 pound Italian sausage
- 2 cups chopped green onions
- 1/3 cup chopped parsley
- 6 ounces black olives, pitted and halved
- salt and pepper to taste

Directions

- ➤ In a blender, combine the oil, vinegar, parsley, salt, sugar, anchovy fillets and garlic. Puree until smooth.

- ➤ Bring a large pot of salted water to a boil. Add potatoes and cook until tender but still firm, about 15 minutes. Drain, cool and cut into cubes.

- ➤ Pour prepared vinaigrette over potatoes and marinate overnight. Place sausage in a large, deep skillet. Cook over medium high heat until evenly brown. Drain, crumble and set aside.

- ➤ Combine the potatoes and dressing, sausage, green onions, parsley and olives. Toss together well and season with salt and pepper to taste.

Roasted Garlic Potato Soup with Smoked Salmon

Ingredients

- 1 whole head garlic
- 2 tablespoons olive oil
- 1/4 cup diced onion
- 1 carrot, finely chopped
- 4 cups chicken stock
- 4 large new potatoes, cut into
- 1/2 inch cubes
- 1/2 teaspoon ground dried rosemary
- 1/4 teaspoon ground thyme
- 3/4 cup heavy cream
- 1/2 cup smoked salmon, torn or cut into bite-size pieces
- salt and pepper to taste
- 1 green onion, thinly sliced

Directions

- Preheat an oven to 375 degrees F (190 degrees C).Cut off the top of the head ofgarlic to expose the cloves, trimming about 1/4 inch off of the top of each clove.

- You may need to trim individual cloves along the sides of the head. Brush the cut cloves with 1 tablespoon of olive oil, then nestle the head into a piece of aluminum foil.

- Bake in the preheated oven until the cloves are tender and nicely browned, about 25 minutes.

- Remove roasted garlic from oven, open foil and allow to cool slightly. When the garlic is cool enough to handle, cut the heads in half horizontally so that all of the cloves are exposed.

- Squeeze both halves to release the roasted cloves into a medium bowl.While the garlic is roasting, heat the remaining 1 tablespoon olive oil in a large saucepan.

- Stir in the onion and the carrot and cook,stirring, until soft, about 5 minutes. Pour the chicken stock into the saucepan and add the potatoes, rosemary, and thyme.

- Bring the soup to a simmer over medium heat and cook until the potatoes are tender, about 20 minutes.

➤ Remove about 1/2 of the potatoes from the pot and reserve. Place the roasted garlic cloves into a blender and add the soup, filling the pitcher no more than halfway full.

➤ Hold down the lid of the blender with a folded kitchen towel, and carefully start the blender, using a few quick pulses to get the contents moving before letting it run. Puree the soup, in batches, until smooth. Pour into a clean pot.

➤ Alternately, you can use a stick blender and puree the soup right in the cooking pot.Stir the reserved potato cubes, heavy cream, and smoked salmon into the pureed soup and bring to a simmer. Serve, hot, with a sprinkle of green onion.

Sweet Potato Rolls

Ingredients

- ❀ 1 (.25 ounce) package active dry yeast
- ❀ 4 tablespoons white sugar
- ❀ 1/2 cup canned sweet potato puree
- ❀ 1/2 cup warm water (110 degrees F/45 degrees C)
- ❀ 3 tablespoons margarine, softened
- ❀ 1 teaspoon salt
- ❀ 2 eggs
- ❀ 3 1/2 cups all-purpose flour

Directions

- ➢ Dissolve yeast, warm water, and 1 tablespoon sugar in a mixing bowl. Let stand 5 minutes. Add remaining sugar, sweet potato, butter or margarine, salt, and slightly beaten eggs. Stir to mix well.

- ➢ Stir in 3 cups of flour. Turn out on a lightly floured surface. Knead 2 to 3 minutes, adding just enough of remaining flour to prevent sticking.

- ➢ Do not knead too heavily; when smooth, shape into a ball. Place in an oiled bowl, and turn to coat the surface. Cover, and let raise about 1 hour or longer.

- ➢ Punch down, and allow dough to rest for 2 minutes. Divide into 16 to 20 balls, and place on a greased cookie sheet or in a 9x13 inch pan. Allow to rise until doubled. Bake at 375 degrees F (190 degrees C) for 12 to 20 minutes. Serve warm.

Whole Wheat Sweet Potato Muffins

Ingredients

- 1 sweet potato
- 2 cups whole wheat flour
- 1 teaspoon baking soda
- 1/2 teaspoon salt
- 1 teaspoon ground cinnamon
- 1/4 teaspoon ground nutmeg
- 1/4 teaspoon ground ginger
- 1/4 teaspoon ground cloves
- 1/4 cup vegetable oil
- 2 eggs, lightly beaten
- 1 teaspoon vanilla extract
- 1 cup honey
- 1 (6 ounce) container vanilla yogurt
- 1/2 cup oatmeal
- 1/2 cup brown sugar
- 1/2 cup almonds
- 1 teaspoon cinnamon

Directions

➤ Preheat an oven to 400 degrees F (200 degrees C). Grease 16 muffin cups, or line with paper muffin liners; set aside. Prick sweet potato several times with a fork and place onto a baking sheet.

➤ Bake the sweet potato in the preheated oven until easily pierced with a fork, about 40 minutes. When the potato is cool enough to handle, peel and mash.Reduce the oven temperature to 350 degrees F (175 degrees C).

➤ Whisk together the flour, baking soda, salt, the 1 teaspoon cinnamon, nutmeg, ginger, and cloves. Stir in the vegetable oil, eggs, vanilla, honey, yogurt, and mashed sweet potato, just until all ingredients are moistened.

➤ Spoon batter evenly into prepared muffin cups. Blend together the oatmeal, brown sugar, almonds, and the remaining 1 teaspoon cinnamon in a food processor or blender. Sprinkle topping over unbaked muffins.

➤ Bake muffins in the preheated oven until golden and the tops spring back when lightly pressed, 12 to 15 minutes.

Rosemary Mashed Potatoes and Yams

Ingredients

- 8 cloves garlic
- 3 tablespoons olive oil
- 1 1/2 pounds baking potatoes, peeled and cubed
- 1 1/2 pounds yams, peeled and cubed
- 1/2 cup milk
- 1/4 cup butter
- 1/2 teaspoon dried rosemary
- 1/2 cup grated Parmesan cheese
- salt and pepper to taste

Directions

- Preheat oven to 350 degrees F (175 degrees C). Lightly grease an 8 inch square baking dish

- Place garlic in small ovenproof bowl, and drizzle with olive oil. Roast for 30 minutes, or until very soft. Cool and peel the garlic, and reserve the oil.

- Boil potatoes and yams in a large pot of salted water until tender, about 20 minutes. Drain, reserving 1 cup liquid.

- Place potatoes and yams in a large bowl with milk, butter, rosemary, garlic, and reserved olive oil.

- Mash to desired consistency, adding reserved cooking liquid as needed. Mix in 1/4 cup cheese. Season with salt and pepper to taste.

- Transfer to the prepared baking dish. Sprinkle with remaining cheese. Bake until heated through and golden on top, about 45 minutes.

Cowboy Mashed Potatoes

Ingredients

* 1 pound red potatoes
* 1 pound Yukon Gold (yellow) potatoes
* 1 fresh jalapeno pepper, sliced
* 12 ounces baby carrots
* 4 cloves garlic
* 1 (10 ounce) package frozen white corn, thawed
* 1/4 cup butter
* 1/2 cup shredded Cheddar cheese
* salt and pepper to taste

Directions

> Place red potatoes, yellow potatoes, jalapeno pepper, carrots and garlic cloves in a large pot. Cover with water, and bring to a boil over high heat.

> Cook 15 to 20 minutes, or until potatoes are tender. Drain water from pot. Stir in corn and butter.

> Mash the mixture with a potato masher until butter is melted and potatoes have reached desiredconsistency. Mix in cheese, salt, and pepper. Serve hot.

Italian Potato Pancake

Ingredients

- 1 medium potato, peeled and grated
- 2 tablespoons chopped onion
- 2 tablespoons whole wheat flour
- 1 egg
- 1/4 teaspoon dried basil
- 1/4 teaspoon dried oregano
- salt and pepper to taste
- 1 tablespoon olive or vegetable oil shredded mozzarella cheese

Directions

- Rinse grated potato in cold water; drain thoroughly. In a bowl, combine potato, onion, flour, egg, basil, oregano, salt and pepper. In a skillet, heat oil; add potato mixture.

- Cover and cook over medium-low heat for 5-7 minutes or until golden brown. Turn; sprinkle with cheese. Cover and cook over low heat 5 minutes longer

Garlic Mashed Red Potatoes

Ingredients

* 8 medium red potatoes, quartered
* 3 cloves garlic, peeled
* 2 tablespoons butter or stick margarine
* 1/2 cup fat-free milk, warmed
* 1/2 teaspoon salt
* 1/4 cup grated Parmesan cheese

Directions

> Place potatoes and garlic in a large saucepan; cover with water. Bring to a boil. Reduce heat; cover and simmer for 20-25 minutes or until the potatoes are very tender. Drain well. Add the butter, milk and salt; mash. Stir in Parmesan cheese.

Italian Potato Salad

Ingredients

- 5 large potatoes, peeled and chopped
- 2 cloves garlic, minced
- 2/3 cup extra virgin olive oil
- 1/2 cup white wine vinegar
- 1/3 cup chopped fresh parsley

Directions

- Bring a large pot of salted water to a boil. Add potatoes and cook until tender but still firm, about 15 minutes. Drain, cool and chop.

- In a large bowl, mix together the garlic, olive oil, vinegar and parsley. Add potatoes and toss to evenly coat.Cover and refrigerate overnight.

Smothered Potatoes

Ingredients

- 5 red potatoes, peeled and cubed
- salt and pepper to taste
- 3/4 cup all-purpose flour for coating
- 1/2 small onion, diced
- 2 tablespoons vegetable oil
- 3 tablespoons water

Directions

- Season potatoes with salt and pepper to taste. Place flour in a shallow dish or bowl; coat potatoes with flour. Add onion to potato/flour mixture and set aside.

- Heat oil in a medium skillet over medium-high heat. When oil is hot add potato/onion mixture and cook until golden brown, stirring occasionally to prevent burning.

- When mixture has browned, reduce heat to low, add water and cover skillet. Simmer for 20 minutes, or until tender.

Potato Pockets

Ingredients

- 4 medium potatoes, julienned
- 3 carrots, julienned
- 1/3 cup chopped red onion
- 2 tablespoons butter or margarine
- 1/2 teaspoon salt
- 1/8 teaspoon pepper
- 1/2 cup shredded Parmesan or Cheddar cheese (optional)

Directions

➤ Divide the potatoes, carrots and onion equally between four pieces of heavy-duty aluminum foil (about 18 in. x 12 in.). Top with butter; sprinkle with salt if desired and pepper.

➤ Bring opposite short ends of foil together over vegetables and fold down several times. Fold unsealed ends toward vegetables and crimp tightly.

➤ Grill, covered, over medium coals for 20-30 minutes or until potatoes are tender. Remove from grill. Open foil and sprinkle with cheese; reseal for 5 minutes or until the cheese melts.

Balsamic Roasted Red Potatoes

Ingredients

- 2 tablespoons olive or canola oil
- 2 pounds small red potatoes, quartered
- 1 tablespoon finely chopped green onion
- 6 garlic cloves, minced
- 1 teaspoon dried thyme
- 1 teaspoon dried rosemary, crushed
- 1/8 teaspoon ground nutmeg
- 1/4 cup balsamic vinegar
- 3/4 teaspoon salt
- 1/4 teaspoon pepper

Directions

- In a large nonstick skillet, heat oil over medium-high heat. Add the potatoes, onion and garlic; toss to combine. Add the thyme, rosemary and nutmeg; toss well.

- Cook and stir for 2-3 minutes or until potatoes are hot. Transfer to a 15-in. x 10-in. x 1-in. baking pan coated with nonstick cooking spray.

- Bake at 400 degrees F for 25-30 minutes or until potatoes are golden and almost tender. Add the vinegar, salt and pepper; toss well. Bake 5-8 minutes longer or until potatoes are tender.

Sweet Potato Bread I

Ingredients

- 1 1/2 cups white sugar
- 1/2 cup vegetable oil
- 2 eggs
- 1 3/4 cups sifted all-purpose flour
- 1 teaspoon baking soda
- 1/4 teaspoon salt
- 1/2 teaspoon ground cinnamon
- 1/2 teaspoon ground nutmeg
- 1/3 cup water
- 1 cup cooked and mashed sweet potatoes
- 1/2 cup chopped pecans

Directions

- Combine sugar and oil; beat well. Add eggs and beat. Combine flour, baking soda, salt, cinnamon and nutmeg. Stir flour mixture into egg mixture alternately with water. Stir in sweet potatoes and chopped nuts.

- Pour batter into greased 9x5 inch loaf pan (or 2 small loaf pans). Bake at 350 degrees F (175 degrees C) for about one hour

Potato Dumplings

Ingredients

- 3 pounds russet potatoes
- 2 eggs
- 1 cup all-purpose flour, divided
- 1/2 cup dry bread crumbs
- 1 teaspoon salt
- 1/4 teaspoon ground nutmeg Dash pepper
- Minced fresh parsley

Directions

- Place potatoes in a saucepan and cover with water; bring to a boil. Reduce heat; cover and simmer for 30-35 minutes or until tender. Drain well. Refrigerate for 2 hours or overnight.

- Peel and grate potatoes. In a bowl, combine the eggs, 3/4 cup flour, bread crumbs, salt, nutmeg and pepper. Add potatoes; mix with hands until well blended. Shape into 1-1/2-in. balls; roll in remaining flour.

- In a large kettle, bring salted water to a boil. Add the dumplings, a few at a time, to boiling water.

- Simmer, uncovered, until the dumplings rise to the top; cook 2 minutes longer. Remove dumplings with a slotted spoon to a serving bowl. Sprinkle with parsley if desired.

Potato Salad Dressing II

Ingredients

- 1/2 cup creamy salad dressing
- 1/2 teaspoon mustard powder
- 2 tablespoons all-purpose flour
- 1 teaspoon butter
- 2 eggs, beaten
- 3/4 cup white sugar
- 1/4 cup water
- 1/4 cup white wine vinegar

Directions

➤ In a saucepan, combine mustard, flour, butter, eggs, sugar, water and vinegar. Cook over medium heat stirring often until mixture becomes thick and smooth.

➤ Remove from heat and allow to cool. Combine dressing mixture with creamy salad dressing, mix well. Fold into cooked potatoes.

Potato Onion Loaf

Ingredients

- 6 baked potatoes
- 2 eggs, beaten
- 1 onion, diced
- 1/2 teaspoon salt
- 1/2 teaspoon white pepper
- 1/2 cup shredded sharp Cheddar cheese

Directions

➤ Preheat the oven to 350 degrees F (175 degrees C). Grease an 8x4 inch loaf pan.Remove skins from potatoes, and discard. Place the potatoes in a large bowl, and mash.

➤ Mix in onion eggs, salt, pepper and cheese with your hands, or as you would meatloaf. Form into a loaf shape and place into the prepared pan.

➤ Bake for 90 minutes in the preheated oven. Let cool for 5 minutes, then remove from the pan, slice and serve.

Sweet Potato Pear Bake

Ingredients

- 1 (15 ounce) can pear halves
- 3 cups cold mashed sweet potatoes
- 4 tablespoons butter or margarine, melted, divided
- 3 tablespoons brown sugar
- 1/4 teaspoon salt
- 1/4 teaspoon ground nutmeg
- 2 tablespoons honey
- 1 tablespoon grated orange peel
- 6 tablespoons whole berry cranberry sauce

Directions

- ➤ Drain pears, reserving 2 tablespoons juice (discard remaining juice or save for another use). In a mixing bowl, combine the sweet potatoes, 3 tablespoons butter, brown sugar, salt, nutmeg and reserved pear juice.

- ➤ beat until combined. Spoon into a greased shallow 1-1/2-qt. baking dish. Arrange pear halves onto top, cut side up.

- ➤ In a small saucepan, combine the honey, orange peel and remaining butter. Cook until heated through. Drizzle half over pears. Bake, uncovered, at 350 degrees F for 30 minutes.

- ➤ Drizzle with the remaining honey mixture. bake 15 minutes longer. Fill pear halves with cranberry sauce

Sausage Potato Bake

Ingredients

- 8 cups cubed potatoes
- 1 pound smoked sausage, sliced
- 1 (10.75 ounce) can condensed cream of mushroom soup
- 1 (10.75 ounce) can condensed vegetable beef soup

Directions

- For oven: Preheat oven to 350 degrees F (175 degrees C).In a 4 quart casserole dish, combine the potatoes, kielbasa OR sausage, mushroom soup and vegetable beef soup. Mix together well.

- Bake at 350 degrees F (175 degrees C) for 1 1/2 hours.For slow cooker: Place the potatoes, kielbasa OR sausage,mushroom soup and vegetablesoup in a slow cooker.Cook on low setting for 6 to 8 hours

Mom's Sweet Potato Bake

Ingredients

- ❀ 3 cups cold mashed sweet potatoes (without added milk and butter)
- ❀ 1cup sugar
- ❀ 1/2cup milk
- ❀ 1/4 cup butter or margarine, softened
- ❀ 3 eggs
- ❀ 1 teaspoon salt
- ❀ 1 teaspoon vanilla extract

TOPPING:

- ❀ 1/2 cup packed brown sugar
- ❀ 1/2 cup chopped pecans
- ❀ 1/4 cup all-purpose flour
- ❀ 2 tablespoons cold butter or margarine

Directions

➢ In a mixing bowl, beat sweet potatoes, sugar, milk, butter, eggs, salt and vanilla until smooth. Transfer to a greased 2-qt. baking dish. In a small bowl, combine brown sugar, pecans and flour; cut in butter until crumbly. Sprinkle over potato mixture. Bake, uncovered, at 325 degrees F for 45-50 minutes or until golden brown.

Creamy Skillet Potatoes

Ingredients

- 7cups cubed uncooked red potatoes
- 1/3 cup chopped onion
- 2 tablespoons all-purpose flour
- 1 (1 ounce) package ranch salad dressing mix
- 1/2 teaspoon dried parsley flakes
- 1/4 teaspoon salt
- 1/4 cup reduced-fat sour cream
- 2 cups fat-free milk

Directions

- Place 1 in. of water and potatoes in a large nonstick skillet; bring to a boil. Reduce heat; cover and simmer for 10 minutes or until tender; drain.

- Coat skillet with nonstick cooking spray; add potatoes and onion. Cook over medium heat for 5-7 minutes or until golden brown.

- In a saucepan, combine the flour, salad dressing mix, parsley and salt. Stir in the sour cream. Gradually add the milk, stirring until blended.

- Bring to a boil; cook and stir for 2 minutes or until thickened. Pour over potatoes; toss to coat.

Zesty Ranch Potato Salad

Ingredients

- ❀ 2 cups Marzetti® Classic Ranch Dressing
- ❀ 4 pounds new potatoes, rinsed, boiled, cooled and quartered
- ❀ 2 bunches green onions, 6-inch section both green and white parts, chopped
- ❀ 4 hard-boiled eggs, peeled and coarsely chopped
- ❀ 1 1/2 cups chopped celery, 1/4-inch pieces
- ❀ 2 teaspoons minced fresh thyme
- ❀ 1 tablespoon minced chives
- ❀ 2 cups coarsely chopped parsley

Directions

➤ In a large bowl, combine all ingredients with Marzetti Classic Ranch Salad Dressing.Toss well and serve. Store remaining portion, covered, in the refrigerator.

Potato Pepperoni Dish

Ingredients

- 2 tablespoons butter or margarine
- 5 large unpeeled potatoes, cut into 1/8 inch slices
- 1 small onion, chopped
- 1/2 teaspoon salt
- 1/8 teaspoon pepper
- 2 cups shredded mozzarella cheese
- 1 (8 ounce) can tomato sauce
- 1 (3.25 ounce) package sliced pepperoni
- 2 large tomatoes, diced

Directions

- ➤ In a 12 in. nonstick skillet, melt butter; remove from the heat. Arrange potatoes on the bottom and up the sides of skillet; sprinkle with onion, salt and pepper.

- ➤ Cover and cook over low heat until the potatoes are tender, about 20 minutes. Sprinkle with cheese; layer with half of the tomato sauce, all of the pepperoni and tomatoes, and the remaining tomato sauce.

- ➤ Cover and cook on low until the cheese is melted and the tomatoes are heated through.

Sour Cream 'n' Chive Potatoes

Ingredients

- 5 1/2 pounds potatoes, peeled and cubed
- 3 teaspoons salt, divided
- 1 cup sour cream
- 1/2 cup milk
- 1/4 cup butter or margarine, cubed
- 1/4 cup minced chives
- 1 teaspoon pepper

Directions

- Place potatoes in a Dutch oven; cover with water. Add 1 teaspoon salt. Bring to a boil. Reduce heat; cover and cook for 20-25 minutes or until potatoes are very tender. Drain well. In a large mixing bowl,

- mash the potatoes, sour cream, milk and butter. Add the chives, pepper and remaining salt; mix well.

Sweet Potato Apple Salad

Ingredients

- 6 medium sweet potatoes 1/2 cup olive or vegetable oil
- 1/4 cup orange juice
- 1 tablespoon sugar
- 1 tablespoon cider or white wine vinegar
- 1 tablespoon Dijon mustard
- 1 tablespoon finely chopped onion
- 1 1/2 teaspoons poppy seeds
- 1 teaspoon grated orange peel
- 1/2 teaspoon grated lemon peel
- 2 medium tart apples, chopped
- 2 green onions, thinly sliced

Directions

➤ In a large saucepan, cook sweet potatoes in boiling salted water until just tender, about 20 minutes. Cool completely.Meanwhile, in a jar with a tight-fitting lid, combine the next nine ingredients; shake well.

➤ Peel potatoes; cut each in half lengthwise, then into 1/2-in. slices. In a 4-qt. bowl, layer a fourth of the sweet potatoes, apples and onions; drizzle with a fourth of the salad dressing. Repeat layers three times. Refrigerate for 1-2 hours. Toss before serving.

Spanish Potatoes\

Ingredients

- 1 1/4 pounds small red potatoes, quartered
- 1 1/2 cups chopped onions
- 1 cup sliced green bell pepper
- 1/2 cup water
- 1 tablespoon olive or canola oil
- 1 teaspoon chicken or vegetable bouillon granules
- 1 cup chopped fresh tomatoes
- 1/2 teaspoon dried oregano

Directions

- Place potatoes in a large saucepan and cover with water. Bring to a boil. Reduce heat; cover and cook for 15 minutes or until tender.

- Meanwhile, in a small saucepan, combine the onions, green pepper, water, oil and bouillon. bring to a boil. Reduce heat; cover and simmer for 8-10 minutes or until vegetables are tender.

- Drain potatoes; add onion mixture, tomatoes and oregano. Stir gently to coat.

Artichoke Mashed Potatoes

Ingredients

- 4 large baking potatoes, peeled and quartered
- 1 (15 ounce) can artichoke hearts in water, drained
- 1 teaspoon minced garlic, or to taste
- 1/2 cup hot milk
- 1/4 cup softened butter
- salt and pepper to taste

Directions

➢ Place potatoes in a large pot with enough water to cover. Bring to a boil over high heat, then reduce heat to medium-low. Cover and simmer until tender, 15 to 20 minutes; drain.

➢ Meanwhile, puree the artichokes and garlic with the milk until smooth. Place drained potatoes in a mixing bowl and mash with a potato masher until smooth.

➢ Stir in softened butter and artichoke puree until the butter has melted. Season to taste with salt and pepper.

Sweet Potato Souffle

Ingredients

- 4 cups mashed cooked sweet potatoes
- 3/4 cup sugar
- 2 tablespoons butter, softened
- 1/3 cup milk
- 1 teaspoon vanilla extract
- 1/2 teaspoon salt
- TOPPING:
- 2/3 cup packed brown sugar
- 2/3 cup chopped pecans
- 2/3 cup flaked coconut
- 2 tablespoons butter, melted

Directions

➤ In a large bowl, combine the sweet potatoes, sugar, butter, milk, vanilla and salt; beat until smooth. Spoon into a greased 2-1/2-qt. baking dish. Combine the topping ingredients; sprinkle over potato mixture.

➤ Bake, uncovered, at 350 degrees F for 40-45 minutes or until heated through and topping is browned.

Mashed Potato Miracle

Ingredients

- 3 cups water
- 1 teaspoon salt
- 5 tablespoons butter
- 2 3/4 cups potato flakes
- 1 onion, minced
- 1 (8 ounce) package cream cheese
- 1 1/2 cups milk
- 1 (6 ounce) can French-fried onions

Directions

- Preheat oven to 200 degrees F (95 degrees C). In a medium saucepan bring water and salt to a boil over medium heat.

- Add butter and stir in potato flakes, onion and cream cheese. Stir in milk until potatoes are soft and fluffy.

- Spoon into a 9x12 inch casserole dish and top with fried onions. Bake in preheated oven for 45 minutes.

Mashed Chipotle Sweet Potatoes

Ingredients

- ❀ 5 1/2 pounds sweet potatoes
- ❀ 1 tablespoon minced chipotle peppers in adobo sauce
- ❀ 3 tablespoons unsalted butter, room temperature and cut into chunks
- ❀ 1 teaspoon salt

Directions

➢ Preheat oven to 450 degrees F (230 degrees C). Lightly grease a 2 quart baking dish, and set aside.

➢ Line a baking sheet with aluminum foil. Pierce each sweet potato several times with a fork, and place on the prepared baking sheet.

➢ Roast the sweet potatoes in preheated oven until easily pierced with a fork, 1 to 1 1/2 hours. Remove from the oven, and cool about 15 minutes.

➢ Reduce oven temperature to 350 degrees F (175 degreesC).When sweet potatoes are cool enough to handle, cut in half, and scoop flesh into a mixing bowl. Discard potato skins.

➢ Beat the sweet potatoes with the chipotle peppers, butter, and salt; spread evenly in the prepared baking dish.

➢ This can baked now orrefrigerated until the next day.Bake in the preheated oven until heated through, 20 to 25 minutes

Skillet Beef and Potatoes

Ingredients

- 3 medium potatoes, halved and cut into 1/4 inch slices
- 1/3 cup water
- 1/2 teaspoon salt
- 1 pound boneless beef sirloin steak, cut into thin strips
- 2 teaspoons garlic pepper blend
- 1/2 cup chopped onion
- 3 tablespoons olive oil, divided
- 1 1/2 teaspoons minced fresh rosemary

Directions

- Place potatoes, water and salt in a microwave-safe dish. Cover and microwave on high for 6-10 minutes or until tender; drain. Season beef with pepper blend.

- In a large skillet, stir-fry beef and onion in 2 tablespoons oil for 5 minutes or until beef is no longer pink.

- Meanwhile, in another skillet, stir-fry potatoes in remaining oil for 5 minutes or until browned. Stir in beef mixture. Sprinkle with rosemary.

Sweet Potato Eggnog Casserole

Ingredients

- ✿ 2 (15 ounce) cans sweet potatoes, mashed
- ✿ 1 cup eggnog
- ✿ 2 tablespoons butter, melted
- ✿ 3/4 cup white sugar
- ✿ 1/2 teaspoon salt
- ✿ 1/2 teaspoon ground ginger
- ✿ 1/4 teaspoon ground cloves
- ✿ 2 tablespoons grated orange zest
- ✿ 1/2 cup chopped pecans

Directions

➢ Preheat an oven to 375 degrees F (190 degrees C). Mix sweet potatoes, eggnog, butter, sugar, salt, ginger, clove, orange zest, and pecans in a large bowl.

➢ Pour into a 2-quart baking dish. Bake in the preheated oven until heated through and golden on top, about 40 minutes.

Striker's Potatoes O'Brien

Ingredients

- 6 large russet (baking) potatoes
- 1 large green bell pepper, cut into 1/2-inch dice
- 1 large red bell pepper, cut into 1/2-inch dice
- 1 large onion, cut into 1/2-inch dice
- 1/4 cup vegetable oil

Directions

- Place the potatoes into a large pot and cover with salted water. Bring to a boil over high heat, then reduce heat to medium-low, cover, and simmer 10 minutes. Drain, then set aside until cool. Once cool, cut into 1/2-inch dice.

- Combine the potatoes, green bell pepper, red bell pepper, and onion in a mixing bowl. Drizzle in the vegetable oil, and gently stiruntil evenly coated. Spoon the mixture into resealable freezer bags.

- Store the mixture in the freezer.To prepare, cook the frozen mixture in a nonstick skillet over medium-high heat until crispy and golden brown, stirring occasionally, about 20 minutes.

Smashed Sweet Potatoes

Ingredients

- ❀ 3 1/2 pounds sweet potatoes
- ❀ 3/4 cup brown sugar
- ❀ 1 orange, zested and juiced
- ❀ 1/3 cup bourbon
- ❀ 1/4 cup butter
- ❀ 1 teaspoon pumpkin pie spice
- ❀ 1 (10.5 ounce) package miniature marshmallows (optional)

Directions

➢ Boil sweet potatoes until tender. Peel and mash until more or less lumpless. Add brown sugar, orange juice and zest, bourbon, butter or margarine, and pumpkin pie spice.

➢ Mix well. Spread in shallow dish (10 inch deep dish pie plate works well). Bake 30 minutes in a 350 degree F (175 degrees C) oven. Top with marshmallows and broil very briefly.

Old Fashioned Potato Kugel

Ingredients

- 1 tablespoon vegetable oil
- 10 potatoes, peeled and grated
- 2 onions, peeled and grated
- 5 eggs
- 1/3 cup vegetable oil
- 2 teaspoons salt
- 1 teaspoon black pepper

Directions

➢ Preheat an oven to 350 degrees F (175 degrees C). Grease a 9x13 inch pan with 1 tablespoon of vegetable oil.

➢ Combine the potatoes and onions in a large bowl. Mix in the eggs, 1/3 cup of vegetable oil, salt, and pepper. Pour the mixture into the prepared pan.

➢ Bake in the preheated oven until the top is golden brown and crisp, 1 1/2 to 2 hours.

Ultimate Twice Baked Potatoes

Ingredients

* 4 large baking potatoes
* 8 slices bacon
* 1 cup sour cream
* 1/2 cup milk
* 4 tablespoons butter
* 1/2 teaspoon salt
* 1/2 teaspoon pepper
* 1 cup shredded Cheddar cheese, divided
* 8 green onions, sliced, divided

Directions

> Preheat oven to 350 degrees F (175 degrees C). Bake potatoes in preheated oven for 1 hour.Meanwhile, place bacon in a large, deep skillet. Cook over medium high heat until evenly brown. Drain, crumble and set aside.

> When potatoes are done allow them to cool for 10 minutes. Slice potatoes in half lengthwise and scoop the flesh into a large bowl; save skins. To the potato flesh add sour cream, milk, butter, salt, pepper, 1/2 cup cheese and 1/2 the green onions.

> Mix with a hand mixer until well blended and creamy. Spoon the mixture into the potato skins. Top each with remaining cheese, green onions and bacon.Bake for another 15 minutes.

Slow Cooker Potato Broccoli Soup

Ingredients

- 4 potatoes, peeled and cubed
- 2 potatoes, peeled and diced
- 1 head broccoli, diced
- 1 onion, minced
- 7 cups milk
- 2 tablespoons garlic powder
- 2 tablespoons minced fresh chives
- 2 cups instant potato flakes
- 1/4 cup dry bread crumbs

Directions

➢ Combine the cubed potatoes, diced potatoes, broccoli, onion, milk, garlic powder, and chives in a slow cooker; cover, and cook on High for 4 hours.

➢ Stir the instant potato flakes and bread crumbs into the soup. Reduce heat to Low and simmer another 30 minutes. Serve hot.

Sweet Potatoes

Ingredients

- ❀ 6 large sweet potatoes
- ❀ 1 (15 ounce) can apricot halves
- ❀ 4 apple - peeled, cored and sliced
- ❀ 1/2 cup packed brown sugar
- ❀ 1/2 cup chopped walnuts
- ❀ 1/2 cup raisins
- ❀ 2 tablespoons butter

Directions

➢ Preheat oven to 350 degrees F (175 degrees C) In a large soup pot, boil potatoes until soft. Add sliced apples just 5 minutes before potatoes are done. Remove from heat. Drain.]

➢ In a large casserole dish, mix potatoes and apples. Dot with butter. Sprinkle brown sugar, walnuts, and raisins on top of potato mixture. Pour apricots over top.Bake uncovered for 30 minutes.

Spanish Potato Salad

Ingredients

- 1 1/2 pounds potatoes
- 8 slices bacon, cooked and crumbled
- 1 small apple
- 1 (2 ounce) can chopped black olives
- 1/4 cup diced red onion
- 1/3 cup white wine vinegar
- 3 tablespoons olive oil
- 2 cloves garlic, minced
- salt to taste
- 1/2 teaspoon ground black pepper

Directions

➢ Bring a large pot of salted water to a boil. Add potatoes and cook until tender but still firm, about 15 minutes; drain and cool. Cut each potato lengthwise into 1 inch spears. Place spears in 9x13 inch baking dish.

➢ Prepare the marinade by whisking together the white wine vinegar, olive oil, garlic, salt and pepper. Reserve 1 tablespoon and pour the remainder over the potatoes and turn gently to coat.

➢ Cover and refrigerate until chilled.Remove potatoes from refrigerator and bring to room temperature.Arrange potato spears on serving platter.

➢ Core apple and finely chop; add to reserved marinade. Stir in bacon (or ham), olives and onion. Spoon over potatoes and serve.

Kartoffel Kloesse (Potato Dumplings)

Ingredients

- 9 medium potatoes, peeled
- 1 teaspoon salt
- 3 eggs, beaten
- 1 cup all-purpose flour
- 2/3 cup bread crumbs
- 1/2 teaspoon ground nutmeg
- 1 cup butter
- 2 tablespoons finely chopped onion
- 1/4 cup dry bread crumbs

Directions

➢ Place the potatoes in a large pot with enough water to cover. Bring to a boil, and cook until the potatoes are soft, about 20 minutes. Drain water, and place potatoes into a large bowl. Mash potatoes, leaving them slightly lumpy (just like making mashed potatoes).

➢ Mix in the salt, eggs, flour, 2/3 cup of bread crumbs, and nutmeg. Roll into walnut sized balls. If the dough is too sticky, you may want to mix in more flour or bread crumbs.

➢ Bring a large pot of lightly salted water to a boil. Gently drop the dumplings into the water. When they come up to the surface, allow them to boil uncovered for 3 minutes.

➢ Remove the dumplings with a slotted spoon, and keep warm. While you are waiting for the water to boil, melt the butter in a skillet over medium heat. Add onions and 1/4 cup of bread crumbs.

➢ Cook, stirring constantly, until the onions are tender, and the sauce has thickened some. Pour sauce over the dumplings before serving.

Whipped Sweet Potato Casserole

Ingredients

- 2 pounds sweet potato, peeled and cubed
- 2 tablespoons orange juice
- 3/4 cup brown sugar
- 1/8 teaspoon ground nutmeg
- 2 tablespoons butter, cubed
- 1 cup miniature marshmallows

Directions

- Preheat oven to 350 degrees F (175 degrees C).In a large saucepan cook sweet potatoes in salted water over medium-high heat for about 20 minutes, or until done.

- Drain, and add orange juice, brown sugar, nutmeg and butter. Whip until smooth. Spread into a medium size casserole dish and top with marshmallows.

- Bake in preheated oven for about 10 minutes, or until marshmallows are golden brown.

Zesty Red Potatoes

Ingredients

- 6 medium red potatoes, halved and thinly sliced
- 1 small onion, halved and thinly sliced
- 1/2 cup butter or margarine, melted
- 1/2 teaspoon crushed red pepper flakes
- salt to taste

Directions

- Arrange potatoes and onion in an ungreased 9-in. square baking dish. Combine butter, pepper flakes and salt; drizzle over potatoes and onion.

- Cover and bake at 400 degrees F for 25 minutes. Uncover; bake 15-20 minutes longer or until potatoes are tender.

Potato Bread I

Ingredients

- 3/4 cup water
- 2/3 cup instant mashed potato
- Flakes
- 1 egg
- 2 tablespoons margarine
- 2 tablespoons white sugar
- 1/4 cup dry milk powder
- 1 teaspoon salt
- 3 cups bread flour
- 1 1/2 teaspoons active dry yeast

Directions

➤ Add ingredients to bread machine in order suggested by the manufacturer.

➤ Add enough water to make a firm dough; use less if leftover potatoes are used. Bake at regular bread cycle

Irish Potato Farls

Ingredients

- ❀ 4 medium potatoes, peeled and halved
- ❀ 1 pinch salt
- ❀ 1/4 cup all-purpose flour, plus extra for dusting
- ❀ 1 tablespoon melted butter

Directions

➢ In a pot, cover potatoes with water and bring to a boil over high heat. Simmer on medium-high heat until the center of the potatoes are tender when pricked with a fork, about 20 minutes.

➢ Turn off heat. Drain, return potatoes to pot and allow to completely dry out over remaining heat.

➢ Mash with a potato masher until smooth. Place warm mashed potato in medium bowl. Stir in flour, salt and melted butter. Mix lightly until dough forms.

➢ On a well floured surface, knead the dough lightly. The dough will be sticky. Use a floured rolling pin to flatten into a 9 inch circle about 1/4 inch thick. Cut into quarters using a floured knife.

➢ Sprinkle a little flour into the base of the skillet and cook the farls for3 minutes on each side or until evenly browned. Season with a little salt and serve straight away.

Light Sweet Potato Casserole

Ingredients

- 3 pounds sweet potatoes, peeled and cut into chunks
- 1/3 cup fat-free milk
- 1/4 cup egg substitute
- 2 tablespoons brown sugar
- 1/2 teaspoon salt
- 1/2 teaspoon vanilla extract
- 1/4 teaspoon ground cinnamon

Directions

➤ Place sweet potatoes in a large saucepan or Dutch oven; cover with water. Bring to a boil. Reduce heat; cover and cook for 25-30 minutes or until tender. Drain.

➤ In a large mixing bowl, beat the sweet potatoes, milk, egg substitute, brown sugar, salt and vanilla until smooth. Transfer to a1-1/2-qt. baking dish coated with nonstick cooking spray.

➤ Sprinkle with cinnamon. Bake, uncovered, at 350 degrees F for 25-30minutes or until heated through.

Kristen's Parmesan Roasted Potatoes

Ingredients

- 1 1/2 pounds unpeeled potatoes, cut into 1-inch chunks
- 2 tablespoons olive oil
- 1 teaspoon kosher salt
- 1/4 teaspoon black pepper
- 1/2 cup grated Parmesan cheese
- 1/4 teaspoon dried thyme leaves

Directions

➤ Preheat an oven to 400 degrees F (200 degrees C).Place the potatoes into a mixing bowl, and drizzle with olive oil.

➤ Sprinkle with kosher salt, black pepper, Parmesan cheese, and thyme leaves. Toss to evenly coat, and transfer to a 9x13-inch baking dish.

➤ Bake in the preheated oven until the potatoes are golden brown on the edges and tender when pierced with a fork, about 1 hour. Serve hot or at room temperature.

Fried Potatoes

Ingredients

- 3 cups diced cooked potatoes
- 1/2 cup diced cooked onion
- 2 tablespoons butter
- salt and pepper to taste

Directions

➢ In a large skillet, cook potatoes and onion in butter over medium heat for 10 minutes or until golden brown. Season with salt and pepper.

Potato and Cheese Pierogi

Ingredients

- 6 cups all-purpose flour
- 3 eggs
- 1 pinch salt
- water as needed
- 5 pounds potatoes, peeled
- 1 pound processed cheese, cubed
- salt and pepper to taste onion salt to taste

Directions

- ➢ Bring a large pot of salted water to a boil. Add potatoes and cook until tender but still firm, about 15 minutes; drain.Combine flour, eggs and salt.

- ➢ Mix in a little water at a time until dough is somewhat stiff. Roll dough in small sections about 1/4inch thick. Using a large biscuit cutter or drinking glass, make circle cuts.

- ➢ To make filling: Mix together potatoes, cheese, salt, pepper and onion salt. Fill each with 1 to 2 tablespoons of the potato mixture, fold over and seal edges.

- ➢ To cook, bring a large pot of water to boil, carefully dropping in one at a time; stir once. They are done when they float to the top.

Asian Potato Salad

Ingredients

- 4 slices bacon, crisply cooked and crumbled
- 6 new red potatoes
- 1 1/3 cups mayonnaise
- 1 teaspoon sugar
- 1 tablespoon soy sauce
- 1 teaspoon sesame oil
- 1/8 teaspoon dry hot mustard
- 1/8 teaspoon salt
- 3/4 cup chopped bok choy
- 1 red bell pepper, seeded and diced
- 1/2 cup chopped green onion
- 1/4 cup chopped fresh cilantro

Directions

- Place bacon in a large, deep skillet. Cook over medium-high heat until evenly brown. Drain, crumble and set aside.

- Meanwhile, bring a large pot of salted water to a boil. Add potatoes and cook until tender but still firm, about 15 minutes. Drain, cool, and chop into bite-size chunks.

- To make the dressing, mix together the mayonnaise, sugar, soy sauce, sesame oil, mustard powder, and salt.

- Combine the potatoes, bacon, bok choy, red pepper, green onion and cilantro in a large bowl. Pour over dressing and mix well. Refrigerate for at least one hour to allow flavors to blend, and serve.

Easy American Potato and Tuna Casserole

Ingredients

- 2 pounds russet potatoes, peeled and cubed
- 1 cup 1% milk
- 4 ounces shredded mozzarella cheese
- 3 tablespoons grated Parmesan cheese, divided
- 2 eggs
- 3 (6 ounce) cans chunk light tuna in water
- 1/2 cup chopped green onion

Directions

➢ Preheat oven to 400 degrees F (200 degrees C). In a large pot over high heat, place the potatoes with water to cover and bring to a boil. Let boil for about 20 minutes, or until potatoes are tender.

➢ Drain and transfer potatoes to a large bowl. Add the milk, mozzarella cheese and 2 tablespoons of the Parmesan cheese. Using an electric mixer, beat the potatoes until almost smooth.

➢ Then beat in the eggs, drain the tuna and stir the tuna into the potato mixture. Then stir in the green onion, and season with salt and pepper to taste.

➢ Transfer mixture to a lightly-greased 10-inch diameter glass pie dish and top with the remaining Parmesan cheese. Bake at 400 degrees F (200 degrees C) for 45 minutes, or until golden brown.

Potato Asparagus Bake

Ingredients

- ❁ 1 pound potatoes, peeled and quartered
- ❁ 1 pound fresh asparagus, trimmed
- ❁ 2 tablespoons butter or margarine, divided
- ❁ 1 tablespoon all-purpose flour
- ❁ 3/4 cup heavy whipping cream
- ❁ 1/2 teaspoon salt
- ❁ 1/4 teaspoon pepper
- ❁ 3 tablespoons dry bread crumbs
- ❁ 3 tablespoons grated Parmesan cheese

Directions

➤ Place potatoes in a saucepan and cover with water. Bring to a boil. Reduce heat; cover and cook for 15-20 minutes or until tender.

➤ Meanwhile, cut the tips off asparagus spears; set aside for garnish. Cut stalks into 1-in. pieces; place in a saucepan and cover with water. Bring to a boil. Reduce heat; cover and cook for 18-20 minutes or until tender.

➤ Drain asparagus and place in a food processor or blender. Cover and process until pureed; set aside. Drain potatoes; mash and set aside.

➤ In a large saucepan, melt 1 tablespoon butter; whisk in flour until smooth. Gradually stir in cream. Bring to a boil; cook and stir for 2 minutes or until thickened. Stir in asparagus pieced, mashedpotatoes, salt and pepper.

➤ Transfer to a greased shallow 1-1/2 quart baking dish. Top with reserved asparagus tips.Melt remain-ing butter; lightly brush some over top.

➤ Toss bread crumbs, Parmesan cheese and remaining butter; sprinkle over casserole. Bake, uncovered, at 350 degrees F for 25-30 minutes or until lightly browned.

Potato Soup III

Ingredients

- 12 potatoes, peeled and chopped
- 1 onion, chopped
- 1/2 pound bacon, cut into small pieces
- 2 1/2 cups milk
- 1 (15.25 ounce) can whole kernel corn (optional)
- 1 1/2 cups dry potato flakes
- 2 cups shredded sharp Cheddar cheese
- 2 tablespoons butter
- salt and pepper to taste

Directions

> In a 3 quart sauce pan, combine potatoes, onion, bacon, and enough water to cover ingredients. Place lid on pot, and cook until potatoes are tender. Stir occasionally to prevent sticking.

> Stir in milk and butter. Stir in instant potatoes to the thickness you desire. Add cheese, and stir until it melts.

> If desired, mix in corn. Season with salt and pepper to taste. Simmer over low heat for 10 to 20 minutes, and serve.

Sweet Potato Fluff

Ingredients

- ❀ 3 cups cooked and mashed sweet potatoes
- ❀ 1 cup white sugar
- ❀ 2 eggs
- ❀ 1/2 cup butter
- ❀ 1/2 teaspoon vanilla extract
- ❀ 1 cup flaked coconut
- ❀ 1 cup packed brown sugar
- ❀ 1/3 cup all-purpose flour
- ❀ 1 cup chopped pecans
- ❀ 1/3 cup butter

Directions

➤ Preheat oven to 350 degrees F (175 degrees C).Mix the mashed sweet potatoes, white sugar, eggs, 1/2 cup of the butter or margarine, vanilla and flaked coconut.

➤ Place in heat proof2 quart sized casserole dish.With a fork mix the brown sugar, flour, pecans and the remaining 1/3 cup of butter or margarine.

➤ Sprinkle over the top of the potato mixture. Bake at 350 degrees F (175 degrees C) for 30 minutes.

Broccoli Potato Bake

Ingredients

- 2 tablespoons butter
- 2 tablespoons all-purpose flour
- 1 teaspoon salt
- 2 cups milk
- 1 (3 ounce) package cream cheese, diced
- 1/3 cup shredded Swiss cheese
- 1 (12 ounce) package frozen hash brown potatoes
- 1 (12 ounce) package frozen chopped broccoli
- 1/2 cup bread crumbs
- 1 tablespoon butter, melted

Directions

➢ Preheat oven to 350 degrees F (175 degrees C).In a large saucepan, melt 2 tablespoons butter. Stir in flour and salt. Add milk and stir until bubbly.

➢ Add cheese, and stir until all of the cheese is melted. Stir in potatoes and heat thoroughly.

➢ Pour half of the mixture into a 10x6 inch baking dish.Cook broccoli according to package instructions; drain well. Layer broccoli over the potatoes in the baking dish.

➢ Pour the remaining potato mixture over the broccoli. Sprinkle the bread crumbs and 1 tablespoon melted butter over the top of the casserole.

➢ Bake at 350 degrees F (175 degrees C) for 20 to 35 minutes; or until bubbly and browned lightly.

Potato-Crust Chicken Quiche

Ingredients

- 4 cups frozen shredded hash brown potatoes, thawed
- 3 tablespoons butter or margarine, melted
- 1 cup shredded Pepper Jack cheese
- 1 cup diced cooked chicken
- 4 eggs
- 1 cup half-and-half cream or milk
- 1/2 teaspoon salt

Directions

➤ Pat hash browns with paper towels to remove excess moisture. Press into a well-greased 9-in. pie plate; brush with butter. Bake at 425 degrees F for 20-25 minutes or until lightly browned. Reduce heat to 350 degrees F.

➤ Sprinkle cheese and chicken into the crust. In a bowl, beat the eggs, cream and salt; pour over chicken. Bake for 20-25 minutes or until a knife inserted near the center comes out clean. Let stand for5 minutes before cutting.

Sweet Potato Pecan Waffles

Ingredients

- 1 cup canned sweet potato puree
- 3 egg yolks
- 1 cup milk
- 1 1/2 cups cake flour
- 1 tablespoon baking powder
- 1 tablespoon white sugar
- 1 teaspoon salt
- 1 teaspoon ground nutmeg
- 1/4 cup chopped pecans
- 3 egg whites
- 3 tablespoons butter, melted
- 2 tablespoons pecans, chopped

Directions

➢ Stir together flour, baking powder, sugar, salt, nutmeg, and 1/4 cup pecans. Mix sweet potato puree, egg yolks, and milk in a large bowl until well combined. Add flour mixture, and mix well. Beat egg whites until stiff peaks form.

➢ Fold 1/4 of the egg whites into batter. Lightly fold remaining whites and melted butter into the batter. Cook in a hot waffle iron. Garnish with more chopped pecans.

Slow Cooker Cream of Potato Soup

Ingredients

- 8 potatoes, chopped
- 3 leeks, white and light green parts only, cut into1/4-inch rounds
- 1 onion, diced
- 3 tablespoons margarine
- 2 chicken bouillon cubes
- 1 tablespoon salt
- 1/2 teaspoon ground black pepper
- 1 (12 ounce) can evaporated milk

Directions

- Place the potatoes, leeks, onion, margarine, chicken bouillon, salt, and pepper in a slow cooker. Pour enough water over mixture to cover.
- Cook on High 4 hours. Stir in the evaporated milk. Ladle soup into a blender and blend until smooth. Serve hot.

Baked Potato Soup IV

Ingredients

- 4 large potatoes, peeled and diced
- 8 cups water
- 1 (12 fluid ounce) can evaporated milk
- 16 ounces heavy cream
- 1/2 cup sour cream
- 3 tablespoons butter
- 1/2 teaspoon onion salt
- 1/2 teaspoon garlic powder salt to taste
- freshly ground pepper, to taste

Directions

➢ Place the potatoes and water in a large saucepan. Bring to a boil. Reduce heat and simmer 1 hour, or until potatoes are very soft.

➢ Mix the evaporated milk, heavy cream, sour cream, butter, onion salt, garlic powder, salt and pepper with the potatoes. Simmer 2 hours, stirring occasionally, until liquid has reduced by 1/3.

➢ Scoop out and drain 1 to 2 cups of the mixture and thoroughly mash with a potato masher. Return to mixture. Garnish and serve.

Grilled Cheese and Bacon Potatoes

Ingredients

- 8 slices bacon
- 4 large baking potatoes, cut into wedges
- 4 (1 ounce) slices processed cheese food
- salt and pepper to taste

Directions

➢ Preheat an outdoor grill for high heat. Place 2 slices bacon each in 4 separate pieces of aluminum foil. The foil pieces must be large enough to fully wrap a potato.

➢ Place one potato in each piece of foil. Top each potato with a slice of processed cheese. Salt and pepper to taste.

➢ Tightly wrap potatoes with the foil. Place on the prepared grill. Cook approximately 30 minutes, or to desired doneness.

Potato and Cauliflower Casserole

Ingredients

- 2 large potatoes, peeled and chopped
- 1 head cauliflower, cut into florets
- 3 tablespoons butter
- 3 tablespoons all-purpose flour
- 1 cup heavy cream
- 1 cup shredded Swiss cheese
- salt and pepper to taste

Directions

- Preheat oven to 350 degrees F (175 degrees C). Lightly grease a medium casserole dish.

- In a pot with enough water to cover, boil the potatoes 10 minutes, or until tender but still firm. Drain, and set aside.

- In a pot, place the cauliflower in a steamer basket over boiling water. Steam 5 minutes, until tender but still firm. Set aside.

- Melt the butter in a saucepan over medium heat, and whisk in the flour. Gradually stir in the heavy cream until thickened. Remove from heat, and mix in 1/2 cup Swiss cheese until melted. Season with salt and pepper.

- Arrange the potatoes and cauliflower in the prepared casserole dish. Pour the cream sauce over the potatoes and cauliflower, and sprinkle with the remaining Swiss cheese.

- Bake 20 minutes in the preheated oven, or until bubbly and lightly browned.

PHILLY Fluffy Mashed Potatoes

Ingredients

- 1 1/2 pounds new potatoes, peeled, cut into chunks
- 1/3 cup PHILADELPHIA Chive and Onion Light Cream Cheese
- Spread

Directions

➤ Cook potatoes in boiling water in large saucepan 20 minutes or until tender. Drain potatoes well; return to saucepan. Add cream cheese spread; mash with potato masher until light and fluffy.

Foolproof Potato Latkes

Ingredients

- 4 potatoes, peeled and cubed
- 1 onion, chopped
- 2 eggs
- 2 teaspoons salt
- 2 tablespoons all-purpose flour, or as needed
- 1 teaspoon baking powder
- 1/4 cup canola oil, or as needed

Directions

➢ Place 1/4 of the potatoes, onion, eggs, salt, flour, and baking powder in the work bowl of a food processor; pulse several times until the vegetables are finely chopped.

➢ Add the rest of the potatoes, and pulse again until all the potatoes are finely chopped and the mixture is thoroughly combined.

➢ Heat canola oil in a skillet over medium heat. Scoop up about 1/3 cup of the potato mixture per latke, and place into the hot oil.

➢ Fry the patty until brown and crisp on the bottom, flip it, and cook the other side until brown, 2 to 3 minutes per side.

➢ Repeat with the rest of the potato mixture, replenishing the oil as needed. Serve hot.

Scalloped Potatoes for the BBQ

Ingredients

- 4 red potatoes, thinly sliced
- 1 large onion, chopped
- 4 cloves garlic, chopped
- 1/4 cup chopped fresh basil
- 1/4 cup butter, cubed
- salt and pepper to taste

Directions

➤ Preheat grill for medium heat.Layer sliced potatoes on aluminum foil with the onion, garlic, basil, and butter. Season with salt and pepper. Fold foil around thepotatoes to make a packet.

➤ Place potato packet on heated grill over indirect heat, and cook for 30 minutes, or until potatoes are tender. Turn over packet halfway through cooking.

Slow Cooker Sweet Potato Casserole

Ingredients

- ❀ 2 (29 ounce) cans sweet potatoes, drained and mashed
- ❀ 1/3 cup butter, melted
- ❀ 2 tablespoons white sugar
- ❀ 2 tablespoons brown sugar
- ❀ 1 tablespoon orange juice
- ❀ 2 eggs, beaten
- ❀ 1/2 cup milk
- ❀ 1/3 cup chopped pecans
- ❀ 1/3 cup brown sugar
- ❀ 2 tablespoons all-purpose flour
- ❀ 2 teaspoons butter, melted

Directions

Lightly grease a slow cooker.In a large bowl, blend sweet potatoes, 1/3 cup butter, white sugar and 2 tablespoons brown sugar. Beat in orange juice, eggs and milk.

➢ Transfer this mixture to the prepared casserole dish. In a small bowl, combine pecans, 1/3 cup brown sugar, flour and 2 tablespoons butter.

➢ Spread the mixture over the sweet potatoes. Cover the slow cooker and cook on HIGH for 3 to 4 hours.

Sweet Potato Pecan Pie by EAGLE BRAND®

Ingredients

- 1 pound yams or sweet potatoes, cooked and peeled
- 1/4 cup butter or margarine
- 1 (14 ounce) can EAGLE BRAND® Sweetened Condensed Milk
- 1 teaspoon ground cinnamon
- 1 teaspoon grated orange rind
- 1 teaspoon vanilla extract
- 1/2 teaspoon ground nutmeg
- 1/4 teaspoon salt
- 1 egg
- 1 (6 ounce) graham cracker pie crust
- PecanTopping:
- 1 egg
- 2 tablespoons dark corn syrup
- 2 tablespoons firmly packed brown sugar
- 1 tablespoon melted butter
- 1/2 teaspoon maple flavoring
- 1 cup chopped pecans

Directions

- Preheat oven to 425 degrees F. With mixer, beat hotyams and butter until smooth. Add sweetened condensed milk, cinnamon, orange rind, vanilla, nutmeg, salt and egg; mix well. Pour into crust.

- Bake 20 minutes. Meanwhile, prepare Pecan Topping, (recipe below).Remove pie from oven; reduce oven to 350 degrees F. Spoon Pecan Topping on pie.

- Bake 25 minutes longer or until set. Cool. Serve warm or at room temperature. Garnish with orange zest twist if desired. Store leftovers covered in refrigerator.

- Pecan Topping: Beat together egg, corn syrup, brown sugar, melted butter and maple flavoring. Stir in pecans.

Bilo Walter's Easy Herb Potatoes

Ingredients

- 2 tablespoons olive oil
- 1 tablespoon balsamic vinegar
- 1 teaspoon garlic salt
- 1 teaspoon dried rosemary, crushed
- 1/4 teaspoon ground black pepper
- 2 small Vidalia onions, wedged
- 3 large carrots, sliced diagonally
- 2 red potatoes, chopped

Directions

➢ Heat a barbeque to a high heat, or preheat oven to 400 degrees F (200 degrees C).In a 9x13 inch baking dish combine olive oil, vinegar, garlic salt, rosemary, and ground black pepper.

➢ Place carrots, potatoes, and onions into the dish and toss to coat.Bake or grill, turning occasionally, until tender (approximately 40 minutes).

Potato Bread IV

Ingredients

- 1 1/8 cups water
- 3 cups bread flour
- 1/2 cup dry potato flakes
- 1 1/2 tablespoons instant powdered milk
- 1 1/2 tablespoons white sugar
- 1 1/2 teaspoons salt
- 1 1/2 tablespoons margarine
- 2 teaspoons active dry yeast

Directions

➤ Place ingredients into the pan of the bread machine in the order suggested by the manufacturer. Select the Basic or White Bread setting. Start.

Blue Cheese Potato Salad

Ingredients

- 4 slices bacon
- 2 pounds red new potatoes
- 1/2 cup olive oil
- 3 tablespoons white vinegar
- 1 bunch green onions, chopped
- 1/2 teaspoon salt
- 1 teaspoon ground black pepper
- 1 1/2 ounces blue cheese, crumbled

Directions

- Place bacon in a large, deep skillet. Cook over medium high heat until evenly brown. Drain, crumble and set aside.

- Bring a large pot of salted water to a boil. Add potatoes and cook until tender but still firm, about 15 minutes. Drain, cool and chop.

- leaving skins on.In a large bowl, whisk together the oil, vinegar, green onions, salt
and pepper. Add the potatoes, bacon and cheese and toss to coat.

The Best Potato Salad

Ingredients

- 6 eggs
- 10 red potatoes
- 1 cup mayonnaise
- 1/2 cup ranch dressing
- 1/3 cup dill pickle relish
- 2 tablespoons prepared yellow mustard
- 1 1/2 teaspoons salt
- 1/4 teaspoon ground black pepper
- 1/8 teaspoon paprika
- 1/8 teaspoon celery seed
- 1 onion, chopped
- 1/4 cup pepperoncini (optional)
- 1/4 cup sliced black olives(optional)

Directions

- Place the eggs into a saucepan in a single layer and fill with water tocover the eggs by 1 inch. Cover the saucepan and bring the water to a boil over high heat.

- Remove from the heat and let the eggsstand in the hot water for 15 minutes. Pour out the hot water; cool the eggs under cold running water in the sink. Peel and chop the cooled eggs.

- Place the potatoes into a large pot and cover with water. Bring to a boil over high heat, then reduce heat to medium-low, cover, and simmer until tender, 15 to 20 minutes. Drain and refrigerate untilcold.

- Peel and cube once cold.Stir together the mayonnaise, ranch dressing, relish, mustard, salt, pepper, paprika, and celery seed in a mixing bowl.

- Add the eggs, potatoes, onion, pepperoncini, and olives; stir until evenly mixed. Cover and refrigerate at least 2 hours before serving.

Yucatan Potato Salad

Ingredients

- 6 russet potatoes, peeled and cubed
- 2 fresh poblano chile peppers
- 3 hard cooked eggs, chopped
- 1/2 cup chopped celery
- 1/2 cup chopped white onion
- 3 medium sweet pickles, chopped
- 12 green olives, sliced
- 1/4 cup lime juice
- 1 cup vegetable oil
- 1 teaspoon salt
- 1/2 teaspoon ground black pepper
- 1 teaspoon mustard powder

Directions

- Preheat the oven to 400 degrees F (200 degrees C). Place the potatoes into a saucepan, and fill with enough water to cover. Bring to a boil and cook until tender, about 10 minutes. Drain.

- Place the peppers into the oven so that they sit directly on the rack. Roast, turning every 10 minutes or so, until evenly charred. Place in a paper bag to sweat, then remove the peel when they are coolenough to handle.

- Remove the stem and seeds, and chop.In a large bowl, combine the still warm potatoes, peppers, eggs, celery, onion, sweet pickles and olives.

- In a smaller bowl, whisk together the lime juice, vegetable oil, salt, pepper and mustard powder.

- I like to use a high speed mixing wand to help it emulsify. Pour over the potato salad, and stir to coat. Adjust seasoning to taste and serve.

Killer Potato Casserole

Ingredients

- 1 (32 ounce) package frozen potatoes au gratin
- 1 (16 ounce) container sour cream
- 4 cups shredded Cheddar cheese
- 2 (10.75 ounce) cans condensed cream of chicken soup
- 2 teaspoons active dry yeast
- 4 cups crushed cornflakes cereal

Directions

- Preheat oven to 375degrees F (190 degrees C).In a large bowl combine the potatoes, sour cream, cheese and soup and mix well.

- Spread mixture into a 9x13 inch baking dish and top with crushed corn flakes Bake for 75 minutes, or until cooked through and golden .

Spicy Glazed Sweet Potatoes and Pineapples

Ingredients

- 3 large sweet potatoes, peeled and cut into 1-inch pieces
- 2 tablespoons ground cinnamon
- 1/2 cup brown sugar
- 1 teaspoon cayenne pepper
- 4 slices bacon
- 1 (16 ounce) can pineapple chunks, drained with juice reserved
- water, as needed
- 1/2 cup sugar
- 1/4 cup brown sugar

Directions

- Preheat oven to 350 degrees F (175 degrees C).Place the sweet potatoes in a saucepan with enough water to cover.

- Add 2 tablespoons cinna-mon; bring to a boil; cook 7 to 10 minutes; drain.Mix together the 1/2 cup brown sugar and cayenne pepper in a small bowl.

- Lie the bacon slices in a baking dish. Sprinkle the brown sugar mix over the bacon.Cook the bacon in the oven until the bacon is crispy, about 10 minutes.

- Place the bacon on a plate lined with paper towels to drain, reserving the liquid from the dish. Change oven setting to Broil.

- Pour the reserved pineapple juice into a measuring cup. Fill the cup with water to measure 1 cup total. Pour the mixture into a skillet and place over medium heat.

- Stir in the sugar, 1/4 cup brown sugar, and 2 teaspoons cinnamon. Cook until the volume of the liquid has reduced to about half. Add the pineapple and drained sweetpotatoes.

- Cook and stir until most of the liquid is absorbed. Transfer the mixture to a round 2-quart casserole dish. Crumble the drained bacon over top of the dish.

- Pour the reserved liquid from the bacon dish over top of the dish.Place the dish under the broiler until the sugar on top caramelizes, 2 to 3 minutes.

Suzy's Mashed Red Potatoes

Ingredients

* 2 pounds small red
* potatoes, quartered
* 1/2cupbutter
* 1/2 cupmilk
* 1/4 cup sour cream
* salt and pepper to taste

Directions

➢ Bring a large pot of lightly salted water to a boil. Add potatoes, and cook until tender but still firm, about 10 minutes. Drain, and place in a large bowl.

➢ Combine potatoes with butter, milk, sour cream, salt, and pepper. Mash together until smooth and creamy.

Swiss Potato Pancake

Ingredients

- 2 tablespoons butter, divided
- 2tablespoons vegetable oil, divided
- 1 (30 ounce) package frozen
  shredded hash brown potatoes, thawed
- 1 teaspoon salt, divided
- 1/4 teaspoon pepper, divided
- 1 1/2 cups shredded Gruyere or Swiss cheese
- Minced fresh parsley

Directions

- In a large nonstick skillet, melt 1 tablespoon butter with 1 tablespoon oil over medium-high heat. Spread half of the potatoes in an even layer in skillet.

- Season with 1/2 teaspoon salt and 1/8 teaspoon pepper. Sprinkle with cheese, then top with remaining potatoes.

- Season with remaining salt and pepper. Press mixture gently into skillet. Cook for about 7 minutes or until bottom is browned.

- Remove from the heat. Loosen pancake from sides of skillet. Invert pancake onto a plate. Return skillet to heat and heat remaining butter and oil. Slide potato pancake brown side up into skillet.

- Cook about 7 minutes longer or until bottom is browned and cheese ismelted. Slide onto a plate. Sprinkle with parsley and cut into wedges.

Parmesan Baked Potatoes

Ingredients

- 6 tablespoons butter or margarine, melted
- 3 tablespoons grated Parmesan cheese
- 8 medium unpeeled red potatoes, halved lengthwise

Directions

- Pour butter into a 13-in. x 9-in. x 2-in. baking pan. Sprinkle Parmesan cheese over butter.

- Place potatoes with cut side down over cheese.Bake uncovered, at 400 degrees F for 40-45 minutes or until tender

Gobi Aloo (Indian Style Cauliflower with Potatoes)

Ingredients

- ❀ 1 tablespoon vegetable oil
- ❀ 1 teaspoon cumin seeds
- ❀ 1 teaspoon minced garlic
- ❀ 1 teaspoon ginger paste
- ❀ 2 medium potatoes, peeled and cubed
- ❀ 1/2 teaspoon ground turmeric
- ❀ 1/2 teaspoon paprika
- ❀ 1 teaspoon ground cumin
- ❀ 1/2 teaspoon garam masala salt to taste
- ❀ 1 pound cauliflower
- ❀ 1 teaspoon chopped fresh cilantro

Directions

➢ Heat the oil in a medium skillet over medium heat. Stir in the cumin seeds, garlic, and ginger paste. Cook about 1 minute until garlic is lightly browned. Add the potatoes.

➢ Season with turmeric, paprika, cumin, garam masala, and salt. Cover and continue cooking 5 to 7 minutes stirring occasionally.Mix the cauliflower and cilantro into the saucepan. Reduce heat to low and cover.

➢ Stirring occasionally,continue cooking 10 minutes, or until potatoes and cauliflower are tender.

Baked Sweet Potatoes with Ginger and Honey

Ingredients

- 9 sweet potatoes, peeled and cubed
- 1/2 cup honey
- 3 tablespoons grated fresh ginger
- 2 tablespoons walnut oil
- 1 teaspoon ground cardamom
- 1/2 teaspoon ground black
- Pepper

Directions

- Preheat oven to 400 degrees (205 degrees C).In a large bowl, combine the sweet potatoes, honey, ginger, oil, cardamom and pepper. Transfer to a large cast iron frying pa Bake for 20 minutes.

- Turn the mixture over expose the pieces from the bottom of the pan. Bake for another 20 minutes, or until the sweet potatoes are tender and caramelized on the outside.

Easy Potato Cheese Soup

Ingredients

- ❀ 8 cups water
- ❀ 6 large potatoes, peeled and sliced paper-thin
- ❀ 1 onion, chopped
- ❀ 4stalks celery, chopped, with leaves
- ❀ salt and pepper to taste
- ❀ 4 cups half-and-half
- ❀ 2 tablespoons margarine
- ❀ 2 (11 ounce) cans condensed cream of Cheddar cheese soup

Directions

➢ In a large stock pot add water, potatoes, onion, celery and season with salt and pepper. Bring to a boil, cover and simmer until potatoes and vegetables are tender.

➢ Once tender, mash soup with a potato masher, and add butter and cream. Gradually bring mixture to a simmer. Add condensed cheese soup and blend. Serve while hot.

Colcannon Irish Potatoes

Ingredients

- 6 medium potatoes - peeled and cubed
- 2 cups chopped cabbage
- 1 large onion, chopped
- 1 tablespoon butter or stick margarine
- 1/2 teaspoon salt
- 1/8 teaspoon pepper

Directions

➢ Place potatoes in a large saucepan or Dutch oven; cover with water. Bring to a boil. Cover and cook over medium heat for 8-10 minutes or until potatoes are almost tender.

➢ Add cabbage and onion. Cover and simmer for 5-6 minutes or until cabbage is tender. Drain well. Mash with butter, salt and pepper.

Cinnamon Sweet Potato Chips

Ingredients   Directions

- ❀ 2 sweet potatoes, peeled and thinly sliced
- ❀ 1 tablespoon melted butter
- ❀ 1/2 teaspoon salt
- ❀ 2 teaspoons brown sugar
- ❀ 1/2 teaspoon ground cinnamon

➢ Preheat oven to 400 degrees F (200 degrees C). Grease two baking sheets. Arrange sweet potato slices in a single layer onto baking sheets.

➢ Stir together butter, salt, brown sugar, and cinnamon in a small bowl; brush onto sweet potato slices.

➢ Bake in preheated oven until edges curl upwards, about 20 to 25 minutes.

Pastetnik Potatoes

Ingredients

- 1 pound potatoes, peeled and cut into 1 inch cubes
- 1/4 cup olive oil
- 1 teaspoon salt
- 1/2 teaspoon ground black pepper
- 1 cup plain yogurt
- 1/3cup mayonnaise

Directions

- Preheat the oven to 425 degrees F (220 degrees C).In a medium bowl, toss potatoes with olive oil to coat, and place in a shallow roasting pan or baking dish. Season with salt and pepper.

- Bake for 1 hour, or until golden brown and tender. Remove from the oven, and transfer potatoes to a large bowl. Stir in yogurt and mayonnaise to coat. Serve immediately.

Potato Chip Cookies V

Ingredients

- 3/4 cup butter
- 3/4 cup white sugar
- 1 egg yolk
- 1 1/2 cups all-purpose flour
- 3/4cup crushed potato chips
- 1/2 cup chopped walnuts

Directions

➢ Preheat oven to 350 degrees F (175 degrees C).In a medium bowl, cream butter and sugar until smooth. Stir in the egg yolk. Add the flour and nuts, mix until well blended.

➢ Stir in the potato chips last, so they don 't get too crunched up. Roll the dough into walnut sized balls.

➢ Place 2 inches apart on an unprepared cookie sheet. Bake for 10 to 12 minutes in the preheated oven. Remove from cookie sheet to cool on wire racks.

Pomegranate Sweet Potatoes

Ingredients

- ❀ 2 sweet potatoes
- ❀ 1/2 cup pomegranate juice
- ❀ 1/4 cup water
- ❀ 2 tablespoons apple cider vinegar
- ❀ 2 tablespoons brown sugar
- ❀ 1/4 teaspoon ground cinnamon
- ❀ 1/4 cup cold butter, cut into tablespoon-sized pieces

Directions

➤ Wrap the sweet potatoes with plastic wrap, and place into the microwave. Cook on High until the sweet potatoes are tender, about 4 minutes, depending on the microwave. Unwrap the potatoes, and refrigerate until cool enough to handle.

➤ Preheat oven to 350 degrees F (175 degrees C). Lightly grease a small baking dish.Bring the pomegranate juice, water, vinegar, sugar, and cinnamon to a simmer in a small saucepan.

➤ Reduce heat to medium-low, and simmer gently for 15 minutes. Meanwhile, peel the potatoes and cut into large cubes; place into the prepared baking dish, and dot with the cubed butter. Pour the pomegranate sauce evenly overtop.

➤ Bake in preheated oven 30 minutes until the pomegranate sauce has thickened into a glaze. Gently stir the potatoes occasionally as they bake to coat them in the glaze.

Baked Sweet Potato Sticks

Ingredients

- ✺ 1 tablespoon olive oil
- ✺ ½ teaspoon paprika
- ✺ 8 sweet potatoes, sliced lengthwise into quarters

Directions

➢ Preheat oven to 400 degrees F (200 degrees C). Lightly grease a baking sheet.In a large bowl, mix olive oil and paprika.

➢ Add potato sticks, and stir by hand to coat. Place on the prepared baking sheet.Bake 40 minutes in the preheated oven.

Gilbert's Potatoes

Ingredients

- 2 1/2 pounds potatoes, peeled and sliced
- 3 onions, sliced
- 1 cup margarine
- 1/2 teaspoon salt
- 1/2 teaspoon ground black pepper
- 6 slices American cheese
- 1 1/2 ounces imitation bacon bits

Directions

➢ Preheat an outdoor grill for medium high heat and lightly oil grate. Use either a 9x13 inch grill-safe baking dish OR a piece of foil large enough to hold all the ingredients.

➢ Layer with the potatoes, onions, pats of margarine, salt and ground black pepper. Sprinkle top with imitation bacon bits. Cover with foil and make sure you seal tightly so the margarine does not escape.

➢ Grill over medium high heat for 45 to 60 minutes, or to desired doneness. Carefully open, arrange the cheese over all and allow a few minutes for the cheese to melt. Remove from grill and serve immediately.

Lime-Thyme Potato Wedges

Ingredients

- ❀ 1/4 cup margarine, melted
- ❀ 1 tablespoon lime juice
- ❀ 1 teaspoon grated lime peel
- ❀ 1 teaspoon dried thyme
- ❀ 3 large potatoes
- ❀ 1/4 cup grated Romano cheese
- ❀ 1/2 teaspoon salt
- ❀ 1/4 teaspoon paprika

Directions

➤ In a large bowl, combine the margarine, lime juice, peel and thyme. Cut each potato into eight wedges; add to lime mixture and toss to coat. Place wedges skin side down on a greased baking sheet.

➤ Combine the cheese, salt and paprika; sprinkle over potatoes. Bake at 400 degrees F for 20-25 minutes or until tender.

Twice-Baked Ranch Potatoes

Ingredients

- 4 large baking potatoes
- 1 (3 ounce) package cream cheese, softened
- 2 tablespoons milk
- 1 (1 ounce) package ranch salad dressing mix
- 1 1/2 cups mashed potatoes
- 1/4 cup shredded Cheddar cheese

Directions

- Scrub and pierce potatoes; place on a microwave-safe plate. Microwave, uncovered, on high for 18-20 minutes or until tender, turning several times. Let stand for 10 minutes.

- Meanwhile, in a small mixing bowl, combine cream cheese and milk; beat in salad dressing mix. Add mashed potatoes; mix well.

- Cut a thin slice from the top of each potato; scoop out pulp, leaving a thin shell. Add pulp to the cream cheese mixture and mash.Spoon into potato shells. Top with cheese.

- Place two potatoes on a microwave-safe plate. Microwave, uncovered, on high for 3-1/2 to 4-1/2 minutes or until heated through. Place remaining potatoes on a baking sheet.

- Freeze overnight or until thoroughly frozen; transfer to a freezer bag. May be frozen for up to 3 months.

- To use frozen potatoes: Place potatoes on a microwave-safe plate. Microwave, uncovered, at 50% powder for 8-9 minutes or until heated through

Potato Soup VI

Ingredients

- 10 pounds peeled and cubed potatoes
- 4 cups non-dairy creamer
- salt and pepper to taste

Directions

➢ Place potatoes in a large pot, and cover with water. The water level should stand about 2 inches above potatoes. Bring to a boil, reduce heat, and simmer until very tender.

➢ Remove soup from heat, and slowly stir in nondairy creamer. Continue stirring until soup is creamy.Mash slightly with a potato masher. Season with salt and pepper. Serve hot or cold.

Sweet Potato Casserole III

Ingredients

- 2 pounds mashed sweet potatoes
- 2 eggs
- 1 1/2 cups white sugar
- 1/4 cup butter
- 1/3 cup sweetened condensed milk
- 1 cup cornflakes cereal, crumbled
- 1/2 cup chopped pecans
- 1/4 cup butter
- 3 tablespoons brown sugar

Directions

➤ Preheat oven to 350 degrees F (175 degrees C). Spray one 2 quart casserole dish with non-stick cooking spray.Combine the sweet potatoes, eggs, white sugar, 1/4 cup of the butter or margarine and the milk.

➤ Mix until well blended. Spoon sweet potato mixture into the prepare casserole dish.Bake at 350 degrees F (175 degrees C) for 15 minutes.

➤ Combine the crushed cornflakes, pecans,remaining 1/4 cup butter or margarine, and brown sugar to taste. Sprinkle over the top of the baked sweet potatoes and return to the oven and bake for another 15 minutes or until lightly browned.

Crispy Mashed Potato Pancake

Ingredients

- ❈ 2 cups cold mashed potatoes (prepared with milk and butter)
- ❈ 1 egg, lightly beaten
- ❈ 1 teaspoon Italian seasoning
- ❈ 1/8 teaspoon garlic powder
- ❈ 1 tablespoon olive or vegetable oil

Directions

➢ Combine the first four ingredients; mix well. In a small skillet, heat oil over medium-high heat.

➢ Add potato mixture; press with a spatula to flatten evenly. Cover and cook for 8 minutes or until bottom iscrispy. Invert onto a serving plate.

Carnation® Creamy Cheesy Mashed Potatoes

Ingredients

- ❋ 2 pounds potatoes, peeled, cut into 1-inch chunks
- ❋ 3/4 cup NESTLE® CARNATION® Evaporated Milk
- ❋ 1/4 cup butter or margarine
- ❋ 1 cup shredded Cheddar cheese
- ❋ 1/8 teaspoon salt, or to taste
- ❋ 1/8 teaspoon ground black pepper, or to taste

Directions

➤ PLACE potatoes in large saucepan. Cover with water; bring to a boil. Cook over medium-high heat for 15 to 20 minutes or until tender; drain.

➤ RETURN potatoes to saucepan; add evaporated milk and butter. Beat with hand-held mixer until smooth. Stir in cheese. Season with salt and pepper.

Spicy Black Bean Potato Salad

Ingredients

- ❀ 8 medium red potatoes
- ❀ 4 eggs
- ❀ 8 slices bacon
- ❀ 1 (15 ounce) can black beans, drained and rinsed
- ❀ 3 green onions, diced
- ❀ 3 fresh jalapeno peppers, diced
- ❀ 1/2 green bell pepper, diced
- ❀ 2 1/2 cups mayonnaise
- ❀ 2 tablespoons brown mustard
- ❀ 1 teaspoon Cajun seasoning
- ❀ salt and pepper to taste

Directions

- ➢ Place potatoes in a pot with enough water to cover. Bring to a boil, and cook until tender. Drain, dice, and cool.Place eggs in a pot with enough cold water to cover.

- ➢ Bring to a boil and immediately remove from heat. Cover saucepan, and let eggs stand in hot water for 10 to 12 minutes. Drain, cool, peel and chop.

- ➢ Place bacon in a skillet over medium-high heat, and cook until evenly brown. Drain, crumble and set aside.

- ➢ In a large bowl, mix chopped eggs, 1/2 the bacon, black beans, green onions, jalapeno peppers, bell pepper, mayonnaise, mustard, and Cajun seasoning.

- ➢ Gently mix in diced, cooled potatoes. Season with salt and pepper, and sprinkle with remaining bacon. Cover, and refrigerate until ready to serve.

Carnation® Mashed Potatoes

Ingredients

- ❀ 2 pounds potatoes
- ❀ 1 cup NESTLE® CARNATION® Evaporated Milk
- ❀ 1/4 cup butter or margarine
- ❀ salt and pepper to taste

Directions

➢ PLACE potatoes in large saucepan. Cover with water; bring to a boil. Cook over medium-high heat for 15 to 20 minutes or until tender; drain.

➢ RETURN potatoes to saucepan; add evaporated milk and butter. Beat with hand-held mixer until smooth. Season with salt and pepper.

Roasted New Potatoes

Ingredients

- ❀ 1 1/2 pounds new potatoes, quartered
- ❀ 2 tablespoons olive oil or vegetable oil
- ❀ 2 garlic cloves, minced
- ❀ 1/2 teaspoon dried rosemary
- ❀ 1/2 teaspoon dried thyme
- ❀ 1/2 teaspoon salt
- ❀ 1/8 teaspoon pepper

Directions

➢ Combine all ingredients in a plastic bag; toss to coat. Pour into an ungreased 13-in. x 9-in. x 2-in. baking pan.

➢ Bake, uncovered, at 450 degrees F for 35 minutes or until potatoes are tender. Remove from the oven and cover with foil to keep warm while broiling the fish.

Sweet Potato Pie I

Ingredients

- 2 1/2 cups mashed sweet potatoes
- 1 2/3 cups evaporated milk
- 1 cup light brown sugar
- 1/2 cup butter, softened
- 2 eggs, beaten
- 1 teaspoon ground cinnamon
- 1 teaspoon vanilla extract
- 1/2 teaspoon salt
- 1/2 teaspoon ground ginger
- 1/2 teaspoon ground nutmeg
- 1 (9 inch) unbaked pie crust
- 1/2 cup all-purpose flour
- 1/2 cup light brown sugar
- 1/2 teaspoon ground cinnamon
- 1/4 teaspoon ground ginger
- 1/4 teaspoon ground mace
- 1/4 pound butter
- 1 1/2 cups sliced almonds

Directions

➢ Preheat oven to 400 degrees F (200 degrees C).Prepare the filling by blending together the sweet potatoes, evaporated milk, 1 cup brown sugar, 1/2 cup butter, eggs,innamon, vanilla, salt, ginger and nutmeg.

➢ Pour filling into prepared crust. Prepare the topping by combining the flour, 1/2 cup brown sugar, cinnamon, ginger and mace. Using a pastry knife, cut the butter into the flour mixture until coarse crumbs form. Stir in nuts.

➢ Sprinkle topping over filling and bake at 400 degrees F (200 degreesC) for 50 minutes or until golden and a knife inserted in the center comes out clean.

Garlic Dill New Potatoes

Ingredients

- 8 medium red potatoes, cubed
- 3 tablespoons butter, melted
- 1 tablespoon chopped fresh dill
- 2 teaspoons minced garlic
- 1/4 teaspoon salt

Directions

- Place the potatoes in a steamer basket, and set in a pan over an inch of boiling water. Cover, and steam for about 10 minutes, until potatoes are tender but not mushy.

- In a small bowl, stir together the butter, dill, garlic, and salt. Transfer the potatoes to a serving bowl, and pour the seasoned butter over them. Toss gently until they are well-coated.

Sweet Potato and Pineapple Casserole

Ingredients

- 1 (29 ounce) can sweet potatoes, drained
- 1 (8 ounce) can crushed pineapple, drained
- 1 tablespoon ground cinnamon
- 1/2 teaspoon ground nutmeg
- 1/2 teaspoon ground cloves
- 15 large marshmallows

➢ Preheat oven to 350 degrees F (175 degrees C).In a large bowl, mash the sweet potatoes until smooth. Add the pineapple, cinnamon, nutmeg and cloves; mix well.

➢ Pour into one 9x13 inch baking dish and top with marshmallows. Bake for 20 minutes or until marshmallows are golden.

Sweet Potato Salad

Ingredients

❀ 2 pounds sweet potatoes, peeled and cubed
❀ 4 tablespoons lemon juice, divided
❀ 2 celery ribs, thinly sliced
❀ 1 (11 ounce) can mandarin oranges, drained
❀ 1 cup fat-free mayonnaise
❀ 2 tablespoons orange juice
❀ 1 tablespoon honey
❀ 1/2 teaspoon salt
❀ 1/4 teaspoon ground ginger
❀ 1/8 teaspoon ground nutmeg
❀ 1/4 cup chopped pecans

Directions

➢ Place sweet potatoes in a large saucepan and cover with water; bring to a boil. Reduce heat. Cover and cook for 9-10 minutes or until tender; drain and place in a bowl. Add 2 tablespoons lemon juice and toss.

➢ Add celery and oranges. In a small bowl, combine the mayonnaise, orange juice, honey, salt, ginger, nutmeg and remaining lemon juice.

➢ Pour over potato mixture and toss to coat. Cover and refrigerate for at least 2 hours. Just before serving, stir in pecans.

Potato Cheese Soup

Ingredients

- 6 potatoes - peeled and cubed
- 1 carrot, chopped
- water to cover
- 3 stalks celery, chopped
- 1 onion, chopped
- 1/2 cup margarine
- 4 cups milk
- salt and pepper to taste
- 2 tablespoons chicken soup base
- 8 ounces processed cheese food, cubed
- 1 tablespoon cornstarch
- 1/2 cup milk

Directions

➤ In a large pot over high heat, combine the potatoes and carrot with water to cover and boil for 10 to 15 minutes, or until tender.In a separate large skillet over medium heat, saute the celery and onion in the margarine for about 10 minutes.

➤ Drain all but about 2 cups of the water from the potatoes and carrots and replace with milk. Reduce heat to low and season with salt and pepper to taste.

➤ Transfer the onion and celery mixture to the pot and stir in the chicken soup base. Heat slowly, then add the cheese. Allow the cheese to melt, stirring all together well.

➤ In a small bowl, dissolve the cornstarch in the 1/2 cup milk and pour into the soup. Mix well until thickened.

Hobo Potatoes

Ingredients

- 4 pounds baking potatoes
- 2 pounds carrots
- 1 onion   seasoning
- salt to taste
- 1/2 cup butter
- 1 1/4 cups sour cream

Directions

➢ Peel and cut up the potatoes and carrots into bite-size chunks. Chop up onion.Combine all veggies in tin foil or foil baking bag.

➢ Season with desired amount of seasoning salt and top with butter. Seal foil well (you may need more than one bag, so the vegetables are done evenly).

➢ Grill for approximately 40 minutes or until potatoes and carrots are soft (flip bags at least 3-4 times during grilling). Remove form grill and place the veggies in a large bowl and add the sour cream,mixing well.

Old-Fashioned Cheese Potatoes

Ingredients

* 1/4 cup all-purpose flour
* 2 teaspoons salt
* 1/2 teaspoon pepper
* 2 1/2 cups milk
* 1 1/2 cups shredded, processed American cheese
* 6 medium potatoes, peeled and thinly sliced
* 1/4 cup butter or margarine

Directions

➢ In a saucepan, melt butter. Add the flour, salt and pepper; cook and stir until a thick paste forms. Gradually add milk.

➢ Cook and stir until the mixture begins to thicken. Add cheese; cook and stir untilmelted. Place potatoes in a greased 3-in. x 9-in. x 2-in baking dish.

➢ Pour sauce over potatoes. Bake, uncovered, at 350 degrees F for 1 hour or until potatoes are tender

Sweet Potato Pie IX

Ingredients

- 3 sweet potatoes
- 1/2 cup butter, softened
- 1 tablespoon vanilla extract
- 2 1/2 cups white sugar
- 1/2 teaspoon ground nutmeg
- 4 eggs, beaten
- 3/4 cup evaporated milk
- 2 (9 inch) unbaked 9 inch pie crusts

Directions

➢ Bring a large pot of water to a boil. Add sweet potatoes and cook until tender but still firm, about 30 minutes. Drain, cool, peel and mash. Preheat oven to 350 degrees F (175 degrees C).

➢ In a large bowl, combine sweet potatoes, butter, sugar, vanilla and nutmeg. In a small bowl, whisk together the eggs and milk and blend into the sweet potato mixture.our into pie shells and bake in preheated oven for 60 minutes, or until done.

Golden Potato Salad with Creamy Harvest

Ingredients

- For the Creamy Harvest Dressing:
- 1 (15 ounce) can sweet potatoes or yams in light syrup, drained
- 1 slice yellow onion, 1/2-inch thick
- 3/4 cup apple juice
- 1/2 cup orange juice
- 1/4 cup red-wine vinegar
- 1/8 teaspoon dried thyme
- 1/4 teaspoon pumpkin pie spice
- 1/2 teaspoon kosher salt
- 1/4 teaspoon freshly ground black pepper
- 2 tablespoons chopped, flat-leaf (Italian) parsley
- For the salad:
- 3 pounds Yukon Gold potatoes, washed, cut in 1 1/2-inch chunks
- 1 small red onion, finely chopped
- 3 ribs celery, peeled and finely diced
- 2 bacon strips, cooked crisp, fat drained and crumbled

Directions

➢ To make the dressing, puree all of the dressing ingredients, except for the parsley, in a blender or food processor until smooth; stir in the parsley.

➢ Boil the potatoes in a large pot of water until tender, about 15 minutes; drain. While still hot toss the potatoes, onion, celery and bacon and the dressing prepared before; set aside to cool.

Zesty Chicken and Potatoes

Ingredients

- 1 cup fat free Italian-style dressing
- 1 teaspoon lime juice
- 1 teaspoon lemon juice
- 1 teaspoon rosemary
- 3 potatoes, chopped
- 2 cloves garlic, quartered
- 5 chicken thighs

Directions

➢ Preheat oven to 400 degrees F (200 degrees C). Lightly grease a medium baking dish.In a bowl, mix the Italian salad dressing, lime juice, lemon juice, and rosemary.

➢ Place potatoes in the baking dish. Distribute garlic evenly throughout dish. Place chicken on top of potatoes. Pour thedressing mixture over the chicken and potatoes.

➢ Seal dish with aluminum foil.Bake 1 hour in the preheated oven, until potatoes are tender and chicken juices run clear.

Pork Chop and Potato Casserole

Ingredients

- 1 tablespoon vegetable oil
- 6 boneless pork chops
- 1 (10.75 ounce) can condensed cream of mushroom soup
- 1 cup milk
- 4 potatoes, thinly sliced
- 1/2 cup chopped onion
- 1 cup shredded Cheddar cheese

Directions

- Preheat oven to 400 degrees F (200 degrees C).Heat oil in a large skillet over medium high-heat. Place the pork chops in the oil, and sear.

- In a medium bowl, combine the soup and the milk. Arrange the potatoes and onions in a 9x13 inch baking dish. Place the browned chops over the potatoes and onions, then pour the soup mixture over all.

- Bake 30 minutes in the preheated oven. Top with the cheese, and bake for 30 more minutes.

Crystal's Awesome Potato Salad

Ingredients

- ❀ 4 potatoes, peeled
- ❀ 1/2 cup chopped onion
- ❀ 1/2 cup chopped celery
- ❀ 2 tablespoons chopped roasted red pepper
- ❀ 2 tablespoons chopped pepperoncini
- ❀ 2 hard cooked eggs, chopped
- ❀ 1/3 cup mayonnaise
- ❀ 1/3 cup sour cream
- ❀ 3 tablespoons dill pickle relish
- ❀ 1 teaspoon Dijon mustard
- ❀ 1 tablespoon prepared yellow mustard
- ❀ 1 clove garlic, minced
- ❀ 1 teaspoon dried dill
- ❀ 1 teaspoon chopped parsley
- ❀ 1/2 teaspoon red pepper flakes
- ❀ salt and black pepper to taste

Directions

➤ Place potatoes in a large saucepan with enough water to cover, and bring to a boil over high heat. Reduce heat to medium low, cover and simmer until potatoes are tender. Drain and cool; cut into 1-inch cubes.

➤ In a large bowl, combine potatoes with onion, celery, roasted red pepper, pepperoncini and eggs.In a small bowl, mix mayonnaise, sour cream, pickle relish, Dijon and yellow mustards, garlic, dill, parsley and red pepper flakes.

➤ Pour mixture over potatoes and stir gently to combine. Season to taste with salt and pepper. Cover and chill for 2 hours before serving.

Taco Potato Pie

Ingredients

- 2 cups cold mashed potatoes (prepared with milk and butter)
- 1 (1.25 ounce) package taco seasoning mix, divided
- 1 pound ground beef
- 1/2 cup chopped onion
- 1 (16 ounce) can refried beans
- 1/2 cup barbecue sauce
- 1/4 cup water
- 1 cup shredded lettuce
- 1 medium tomato, seeded and chopped
- 1 cup shredded Cheddar cheese Sour cream

Directions

➢ Combine the potatoes and 2 tablespoons taco seas-oning. Press into a greased 9-in. deep-dish pie plate; set aside.

➢ In a skillet, cook beef and onion over medium heat until meat is no longer pink; drain. Stir in the beans, barbecue sauce, water and remaining taco seasoning. Cook and stir until hot and bubbly. Spoon into potato crust.

➢ Bake at 350 degrees F for 30-35 minutes or until heated through. Top with lettuce, tomato, cheese and sour cream.

Savory Kale, Cannellini Bean, and Potato Soup

Ingredients

- ❀ 2 tablespoons extra-virgin olive oil
- ❀ 1 onion, diced
- ❀ 3/4 cup diced carrot
- ❀ 4 cloves garlic, minced
- ❀ 3 cups low-sodium chicken broth
- ❀ 2 cups water
- ❀ 1 cup white wine
- ❀ 3 potatoes, halved and sliced
- ❀ 1/2 teaspoon chopped fresh rosemary
- ❀ 1/2 teaspoon chopped fresh sage
- ❀ 1/2 teaspoon chopped fresh
- ❀ thyme
- ❀ 1 (16 ounce) can cannellini beans, rinsed and drained
- ❀ 2 cups finely chopped kale leaves
- ❀ 1 small red chile pepper, seeded and chopped fine
- ❀ ground black pepper to taste

Directions

➢ Heat the olive oil in a large Dutch oven over medium heat; cook and stir the onion until softened and transl-ucent, about 5 minutes. Stir in the carrot and garlic, and cook for 5 minutes more.

➢ Pour in the chicken broth, water, and white wine; stir in the potatoes, rosemary, sage, and thyme. Bring to a boil over high heat, then reduce heat to medium-low, cover, and simmer until the potatoes are tender, about 20 minutes.

➢ Add the cannelini beans, kale, chile pepper, and black pepper, and simmer, covered, for 30 more minutes.

Sweet Potato Salad

Ingredients

- 2 pounds sweet potatoes, peeled and cubed
- 1 cup mayonnaise
- 1/2 cup packed brown sugar
- 1 cup chopped walnuts
- 1/2 cup raisins

Directions

➢ Place potatoes into a large saucepan, and fill with enough water to cover. Bring to a boil, and cook for about 8 minutes, or until tender. Drain, and cool slightly.

➢ In a large bowl, stir together the mayonnaise and brown sugar. Stir in the sweet potatoes, walnuts and raisins until evenly coated. Chill for at least 1 hour before serving.

Microwave German Potato Salad

Ingredients

- ❀ 2 pounds red potatoes, cooked and sliced
- ❀ 3 hard-cooked eggs, chopped
- ❀ 1/2 cup chopped onion
- ❀ 1/2 cup chopped celery
- ❀ 6 bacon strips, diced
- ❀ 2 tablespoons sugar
- ❀ 4 teaspoons all-purpose flour
- ❀ 2 tablespoons vinegar
- ❀ 1/2 teaspoon salt
- ❀ 1/8 teaspoon pepper
- ❀ 3/4 cup milk

Directions

➢   In a large bowl, combine potatoes, eggs, onion and celery; set aside. Place bacon in a microwave-safe bowl; cover with a paper towel and microwave on high for 2 minutes.

➢ Stir Microwave 3-4minutes longer or until the bacon is crisp, stirring after each minute. Remove bacon to paper towel to drain; reserve 2 tablespoons drippings.

➢ Stir sugar, flour, vinegar, salt and pepper into drippings until smooth; gradually add milk. Microwave on high for 5-6 minutes, stirring every 2 minutes until thickened. Pour over potato mixture; toss. Top with bacon. Serve immediately.

Creamy Irish Potato Soup

Ingredients

- ❀ 2 tablespoons butter or margarine
- ❀ 4 green onions, sliced
- ❀ 1 stalk celery, sliced
- ❀ 1 3/4 cups SwansonB® Chicken Broth (regular, Natural Goodnessʙ „ў or Certified Organic)
- ❀ 1/8 teaspoon ground black pepper
- ❀ 3 medium potatoes, peeled and sliced 1/4 inch thick
- ❀ 1 1/2 cups milk

Directions

➢ Heat butter in saucepan. Add onions and celery and cook until tender. Add broth, black pepper and potatoes. Heat to a boil. Cover and cook over low heat 15 minutes or until potatoes are tender.

➢ Place half the broth mixture and half the milk in blender or food processor. Cover and blend until smooth. Repeat with remaining broth mixture and remaining milk. Return to saucepan. Heat through.

Easy Sweet Potatoes with Kahlua

Ingredients

- 4 large sweet potatoes, peeled and cubed
- 1/2 cup butter
- 2/3 cup brown sugar
- 1/2 cup coffee flavored liqueur (such as Kahlua®)
- 1/4 cup raisins (optional)
- 1/4 cup toasted pecans (optional)

Directions

> Place the sweet potatoes into a large pot and cover with salted water. Bring to a boil over high heat, then reduce heat to medium-low, cover, and simmer until tender, about 20 minutes.

> Drain and allow to steam dry for a minute or two. Return the pot to the stove over medium heat. Add the butter and brown sugar; cook and stir about 5 minutes until the sugar begins to caramelize.

> The sugar will be foamy at first, then the foam will subside and the sugar will begin to caramelize; cook until the color darkens slightly.

> Carefully stir in the coffee liqueur, then return the potatoes to the pot. Stir in the raisins and toasted pecans until the potatoes are slightly mashed and everything is well mixed.

Potato Scones

Ingredients

- 2 cups all-purpose flour
- 1 tablespoon baking powder
- 1 teaspoon salt
- 3 tablespoons cold butter or margarine
- 1 cup mashed potatoes (prepared with milk and butter)
- 1/3 cup milk
- 1 egg

Directions

➢ In a bowl, combine the flour, baking powder and salt. Cut in butter until mixture resembles coarse crumbs. Combine potatoes, milk and egg; stir into the crumb mixture until a soft dough forms.

➢ Turn onto a floured surface; knead gently 10-12 minutes or until no longer sticky. Gently pat or roll dough into a 9-in. circle about 3/4 in. thick. Cut into 10-12 wedges.

➢ Separate wedges and place on an ungreased baking sheet. Bake at 400 degrees F for 15-18 minutes or until golden brown.

Leftover Scalloped Potato Soup

Ingredients

- 4 cups leftover scalloped potatoes
- 4 cups chicken broth, or as needed
- 1 tablespoon garlic powder salt and pepper to taste
- 1 cup cubed cooked ham (optional)
- 1 cup shredded Cheddar cheese
- 1/4 cup grated Parmesan cheese

Directions

- Place the scalloped potatoes into a large pot, and pour in enough chicken broth to cover the potatoes completely. Season with garlic powder, salt and pepper.

- Add ham if using. Bring to a boil, and reduce heat to low. Stir in the Cheddar and Parmesan cheese, and simmer for about 10 minutes.

Onion Potato Rolls

Ingredients

- 2 (.25 ounce) packages active dry yeast
- 1/2 cup warm water (110 degrees F to 115 degrees F)
- 1 cup warm milk (110 to 115 degrees F)
- 1 cup mashed potato flakes
- 1/2 cup butter or margarine, softened
- 1/2 cup packed brown sugar
- 2 eggs
- 1 envelope onion soup mix
- 1 teaspoon salt
- 2 cups whole wheat flour
- 2 1/2 cups all-purpose flour TOPPING:
- 1 egg
- 1/4 cup dried minced onion

Directions

➢ In a mixing bowl, dissolve yeast in warm water. Add the next eight ingredients; mix well. Stir in enough all-purpose flour to form a soft dough. Turn onto a floured surface; knead until smooth and elastic, about 6-8 minutes. Place in a greased bowl, turning once to grease top.

➢ Cover and let rise in a warm place until doubled, about 1 hour. Punch the dough down; divide into 18 pieces. Shape each into a ball.

➢ Place 2 in. apart on greased baking sheets. Cover and let rise until doubled, about 30 minutes. Beat egg; brush over rolls. Sprinkle with dried onion. Bake at 350 degrees F for 15-18 minutes or until golden brown. Remove to wire racks to cool.

Black Bean, Sausage, and Sweet Potato Soup

Ingredients

- 5 1/2 cups water
- 1 1/2 cups dry black beans
- 3 cloves garlic, minced
- 1 bay leaf
- 1/4 teaspoon ground allspice
- 2 cups chicken broth
- 1 tablespoon tomato paste
- 1 tablespoon water
- 1/4 pound Italian sausage, cut into 1/2 inch pieces
- ½ teaspoon Worcestershire sauce
- 1 pound sweet potatoes
- 3 green onions
- salt to taste ground black pepper to taste

Directions

➢ In a 4 quart saucepan, combine beans, garlic, bay leaf, allspice, broth and 5 1/2 cups water. Cook, partially covered, until beans are tender, about 50 minutes. Discard bay leaf.

➢ In a blender puree 1 cup cooked beans with 1 cup cooking liquid, and return to pan.

➢ In a small bowl, stir together tomato paste and 1 tablespoon water; stir into beans with sausage and Worcestershire sauce. Simmer soup, covered, for 15 minutes. Soup may be prepared up to this point 3 days ahead.

➢ While soup is simmering, peel sweet potatoes and cut into 1/2 inch pieces. Steam until tender, about 10 minutes. Stir potatoes, 3 chopped scallions, and salt and pepper to taste into soup. Serve soup garnished with scallion greens.

Orange Glazed Sweet Potatoes

Ingredients

- 6 sweet potatoes
- 3/4 cup boiling water
- 1 teaspoon salt
- 3 tablespoons butter
- 1/2 tablespoon orange zest
- 1 tablespoon orange juice
- 3/4 cup light corn syrup
- 1/4 cup packed brown sugar
- 3 orange slices, halved

Directions

➢ Pare and halve sweet potatoes. Combine peel, juice, corn syrup, and brown sugar. Add sweet potatoes, boiling water, and salt to a large saucepan.

➢ Simmer, cove-red, until tender; this should take about 15 minutes. Drain off liquid, leaving 1/4 cup in skillet. Dot potatoes with butter or margarine.

➢ Pour orange juice mixture over potatoes, and add orange slices. Cook, uncovered, over low heat until glazed, an additional 15 minutes. Baste often, and turn once while cooking.

Asparagus, Potato, and Onion Frittata

Ingredients

- 2 tablespoons olive oil
- 2potatoes, shredded
- 1/4 cup chopped onion
- 1/2 teaspoon salt
- 1/4 teaspoon fresh ground black pepper
- 1 pound asparagus, trimmed and cut into 2-inch pieces
- 1 cup diced ham
- 6 eggs
- 1 tablespoon milk
- 1/2 cup shredded mozzarella cheese
- 1/2 cup shredded white Cheddar cheese
- 1 tablespoon chopped fresh basil

Directions

- Preheat an oven to 350 degrees F (175 degrees C). Grease a 9x13 inch baking dish.

- Heat the olive oil in a large skillet over medium heat; cook and stir the shredded potato and onion in the hot oil until the potatoes begin to brown, about 5 minutes.. Season with salt and pepper.

- Add the asparagus and ham and continue cooking until the asparagus is tender, another 5 to 7 minutes; transfer to the prepared baking dish.

- Whisk the eggs and milk together in a small bowl; pour evenly over the dish. Scatter the mozzarella and white Cheddar cheeses over the top of the potato mixture.

- Bake in the preheated oven until set in the middle, 20 to 25 minutes. Garnish with the basil to serve.

Hot German Potato Salad

Ingredients

- 8 medium potatoes, cut into 1/4-inch slices
- 2 celery ribs, chopped
- 1 large onion, chopped
- 1 cup water
- 2/3 cup cider vinegar
- 1/3 cup sugar
- 2 tablespoons quick-cooking tapioca
- 1 teaspoon salt
- 3/4 teaspoon celery seed
- 1/4 teaspoon pepper
- 6 bacon strips, cooked and crumbled
- 1/4 cup minced fresh parsley

Directions

➢ In a slow cooker, combine potatoes, celery and onion. In a bowl, combine water, vinegar, sugar, tapioca, salt, celery seed and pepper.

➢ Pour over potatoes; stir gently to coat. Cover and cook on high for 4-5 hours or until potatoes are tender. Just before serving, sprinkle with bacon and parsley

Sweet Potato Loaves

Ingredients

- 1/4 cup butter or margarine, softened
- 1/2 cup sugar
- 1 egg
- 1 cup all-purpose flour
- 1 1/2 teaspoons baking powder
- 1/2 teaspoon ground cinnamon
- 1/4 teaspoon ground ginger
- 1/4 teaspoon salt
- 1/2 cup cold mashed sweet potatoes
- 2 tablespoons milk
- 1/4 cup raisins

Directions

➢ In a small mixing bowl, cream butter and sugar. Add egg; mix well. Combine the flour, baking powder, cinnamon, ginger and salt; add to creamed mixture just until blended (batter will be thick).

➢ Combine sweet potatoes and milk; stir into batter until blended. Fold in raisins. Transfer to two greased 5-3/4-in. x 3-in. x 2-in. loaf pans.

➢ Bake at 350 degrees F for 35-40 minutes or until lightly browned and a toothpick inserted near the center comes out clean. Cool for 10 minutes before removing from pans to wire racks.

Hot German Potato Salad II

Ingredients

- 3 pounds potatoes
- 1 pound bacon, cubed
- 1 onion, diced
- 2 cups white sugar
- 2 cups white wine vinegar

Direction

- Bring a large pot of salted water to a boil. Add potatoes and cook until tender but still firm, about 15 minutes. Drain, cool and chop.

- Place bacon and onion in a large, deep skillet. Cook over medium heat until bacon is evenly brown. Drain excess grease from skillet.

- Add the sugar and vinegar to the bacon and onion mixture and bring to a boil. Pour the mixture over the potatoes and stir.

Dijon Mashed Potatoes

Ingredients

- 3 large potatoes, peeled and cubed
- 3/4 cup reduced fat sour cream
- 1/2 cup nonfat milk
- 2 tablespoons Dijon mustard garlic salt to taste
- ground black pepper to taste

Directio

- Place the cubed potatoes in a pot with enough water to cover. Bring to a boil, and cook 15 minutes, or until tender.

- Drain potatoes and transfer to a bowl. Mash with a potato masher, and gradually mix in the sour cream, nonfat milk, and Dijon mustard. Season with garlic salt and pepper.

Dressing for Potato Salad

Ingredients

- 1/2 cup mayonnaise
- 1/2 cup sour cream
- 2 teaspoons prepared mustard
- 1 tablespoon ketchup
- 1 1/2 teaspoons Worcestershire sauce
- 1/2 cup diced onion (optional) salt and pepper to taste

Directions

- Mix together the mayon-naise, sour cream, mustard, ketchup, Worce-stershire sauce, onion and salt and pepper. Refrigerate until ready to toss with potatoes.

Potato Chip Crunchies

Ingredients

- 2 cups butter, softened
- 1 1/2 cups sugar
- 1 egg
- 1 teaspoon vanilla extract
- 4 cups all-purpose flour
- 1 cup crushed potato chips
- 1 cup chopped pecans

Directions

- In a mixing bowl, cream butter and sugar. Beat in egg and vanilla. Gradually add flour. Fold in the potato chips and pecans. Drop by tablespoonfuls 1-1/2 in. apart onto ungreased baking sheets.

- Flatten with a fork. Bake at 350 degrees F for 12-14 minutes or until golden brown. Remove to wire racks to cool.

Potatoes Madras

Ingredients

- 3 tablespoons vegetable oil
- 1 1/2 pounds potatoes, cut into 1/2 inch dice
- 2 1/2 cups cauliflower florets
- 1 large onion, sliced
- 2 cloves garlic, crushed
- 1 tablespoon curry powder
- 1/2 tablespoon ground ginger
- 4 ounces dry red lentils
- 1 (14.4 ounce) can whole tomatoes, chopped
- 1 1/4 cups vegetable stock
- 2 tablespoons malt vinegar
- 1 tablespoon mango chutney
- salt and pepper to taste
- chopped fresh parsley for garnish

Directions

> Warm oil in a large skillet over medium heat. Stir in potatoes, cauliflower, onion, and garlic; cook until the garlic begins to brown. Stir in the curry powder and ginger, and cook about 3 minutes.

> Stir in lentils, tomatoes, vegetable stock, vinegar, and chutney. Season with salt and pepper. Cover, and simmer, stirring occasionally, until the lentils are tender, about 20 minutes. Top with parsley.

Picnic Celery and Potato Salad

Ingredients

- ❀ 10 medium red potatoes, cut into 1-inch pieces
- ❀ 1 (10.75 ounce) can Campbell's® Condensed Cream of Celery Soup (Regular or 98% Fat Free)
- ❀ 2 tablespoons prepared mustard
- ❀ 2 tablespoons lemon juice
- ❀ 1 tablespoon cider vinegar
- ❀ 1/4 teaspoon prepared Horseradish
- ❀ 4 stalks celery, chopped
- ❀ 1 small onion, chopped Ground black pepper

Directions

- ➢ Place the potatoes into a 6-quart saucepot and add water to cover. Heat over medium-high heat to a boil. Reduce the heat to low. Cook for 10 minutes or until the potatoes are tender. Drain the potatoes well in a colander.

- ➢ Stir the soup, mustard, lemon juice, vinegar and horseradish in a large bowl. Add the potatoes, celery and onion and toss to coat. Season with the black pepper. Cover and refrigerate for 2 hours.

Delmonico Potatoes

Ingredients

- 1 (2 pound) package frozen hash brown potatoes, thawed
- 1 (8 ounce) package processed cheese
- 2 cups half-and-half
- 1/2 cup butter

Directions

- Preheat oven to 350 degrees F (175 degrees C). Place frozen potatoes in a 13 x 9 inch baking dish.

- In a saucepan on the stovetop or in microwave on low, melt together cheese and butter or margarine. When melted, blend in the cream.

- Pour mixture over frozen potatoes, and cover pan with foil. Bake for 1 hour. Remove foil, and bake 15 minutes more.

Potato Casserole II

Ingredients

- 3 1/2 cups instant mashed potato flakes
- 3/4 cup sour cream
- 1 (3 ounce) can bacon bits
- 1 pound mild Cheddar cheese

Directions

➢ Preheat oven to 350 degrees F (175 degrees C). Prepare potatoes according to package directions. Add sour cream and bacon bits; mix well.

➢ Place in a 9x13 inch baking dish and top with cheese; bake for 30 minutes or until cheese is melted.

Cheesy Potato Bread

Ingredients

- 2 (.25 ounce) packages active dry yeast
- 2 tablespoons sugar
- 1/2 cup warm water (110 degrees F to 115 degrees F)
- 1 cup half-and-half cream
- 5 tablespoons butter or margarine, melted, divided
- 1 tablespoon salt
- 1/8 teaspoon cayenne pepper
- 5 1/2 cups all-purpose flour
- 2 cups finely shredded peeled potatoes
- 1 cup shredded Cheddar cheese

Directions

➢ In a large mixing bowl, dissolve the yeast and sugar in warm water; let stand until foamy, about 5 minutes. Add cream, 3 tablespoons butter, salt, cayenne pepper and 2-1/2 cups flour; beat on medium for 2 minutes.

➢ Stir in potatoes and enough remaining flour to form a soft dough. Turn onto a floured surface; knead until smooth and elastic, about 8-10 minutes. (Dough will feel slightly sticky.)

➢ Place in a greased bowl, turning once to grease top. Cover and let rise in a warm place until almost doubled, about 1 hour. Punch the dough down. Pat into a 1/2-in.-thick rectangle.

➢ Sprinkle cheese evenly over dough. Fold dough over the cheese and knead into dough. Shape into two round loaves; place in greased 9-in. round baking pans.

➢ Cover and let rise until doubled, about 45 minutes. Cut an X on top of each loaf; brush with remaining butter. Bake at 400 degrees F for 35-40 minutes or until golden brown. Remove from pans to cool on wire racks.

Cinnamon Pork Loin and Potatoes

Ingredients

* ❀ 2 pounds boneless pork loin roast
* ❀ 4 red potatoes, peeled and sliced
* ❀ salt and pepper to taste
* ❀ 3 sweet potatoes, peeled and sliced
* ❀ 2 tablespoons ground cinnamon
* ❀ 1 tart green apple - peeled, cored, and sliced
* ❀ 1/2 cup butter, sliced
* ❀ 1/2 cup milk
* ❀ 1/2 cup water
* ❀ 2 cubes chicken bouillon
* ❀ 1 cube beef bouillon
* ❀ 1 tablespoon cornstarch

Directions

➤ Preheat oven to 375 degrees F (190 degrees C). Place the pork roast in a medium baking dish. Season red potatoes with salt and pepper, and arrange around the roast.

➤ Place sweet potatoes and cinnamon in a resealable plastic bag, and shake to
coat. Arrange sweet potatoes around the roast. Place apple over the roast and potatoes. Top with butter slices. Seal baking dish tightly with foil.

➤ Cook 1 1/2 hours in the preheated oven, or until the internal temperature of the pork has reached 160 degrees F (70 degrees C).

➤ In a medium saucepan over medium heat, blend the milk, water, chicken bouillon, beef bouillon, and cornstarch until the bouillon cubes are dissolved and the mixture is thickened. Serve with the pork roast and potatoes.

Potato Pancakes II

Ingredients

- 2 cups mashed potatoes
- 1 egg, beaten
- 1 teaspoon salt
- 1/4 cup shredded Cheddar cheese
- 1 tablespoon butter

Directions

➤ In a medium bowl, mix together potatoes, beaten egg, salt, and cheese. Melt butter on a large griddle at medium heat. Drop potato mixture onto griddle 1/4 cup at a time.

➤ Flatten with a spatula to 1/2 inch thick. Fryapproximately 5 minutes on each side, until golden brown. Serve hot.

Parsley Potatoes

Ingredients

- 1 1/2 pounds new red potatoes
- 1 tablespoon vegetable oil
- 1 onion, chopped
- 1 clove garlic, crushed
- 1 cup chicken broth
- 1 cup chopped fresh parsley
- 1/2 teaspoon ground black pepper

Directions

- ➤ Peel a strip of skin from around the center of each potato, place the potatoes in cold water. Set aside.

- ➤ Heat oil in a large skillet over medium high heat. Saute onion and garlic for 5 minutes or until tender. Pour in broth and 3/4 cup of the parsley; mix well. Bring to a boil.

- ➤ Place the potatoes into a large pot full of salted water. Bring the water to a boil; then reduce heat. Simmer covered, for 10 minutes or until the potatoes are tender.

- ➤ Remove potatoes with a slotted spoon to a serving bowl. Sprinkle the black pepper into the skillet and stir.. Pour the peppered sauce over potatoes and sprinkle with remaining parsley.

Quick and Easy Ham with Sweet Potatoes

Ingredients

- 2 ham steaks
- 1/4 cup packed brown sugar
- 1 (8 ounce) can crushed pineapple, drained
- 1 (15 ounce) can sweet potatoes, drained
- 1 cup miniature marshmallows

Directions

- Preheat the oven to 350 degrees F (175 degrees C). Tear off two large sheets of aluminum foil. Place one ham slice onto each piece of foil, and sprinkle brown sugar on both sides.

- Spread a little bit of the crushed pineapple over the ham, then top with sweet potatoes. Sprinkle a little bit more brown sugar and pineapple over the sweet potatoes. Close the aluminum foil tightly around the ham, and place on a baking sheet.

- Bake for 30 minutes in the preheated oven. Remove from the oven, and carefully open the packets. Sprinkle miniaturemarshmallows over the top, and return to the oven with the foil open.

- Bake for another 10 minutes. If you want the marshmallows really toasty, you could brown them under the broiler for a couple of minutes. You will end up with a sweet, juicy ham dish and very few dishes to wash.

Syracuse Salt Potatoes

Ingredients

- 4 pounds new potatoes
- 1 1/2 cups fine salt
- 8 tablespoons butter, melted

Directions

➤ Wash the potatoes and set aside. Fill a large pot with water; stir in salt until it no longer dissolves and settles on the bottom.

➤ Place potatoes in the pot and bring to a boil; reduce heat and simmer until potatoes are tender but firm, about 15 minutes. Drain; cover to keep hot.

➤ While the potatoes are cooking, melt the butter in a small pan over medium high heat, or in microwave. Serve immediately poured over potatoes.

Sausage, Peppers, Onions, and Potato Bake

Ingredients

- ❀ 2 teaspoons olive oil
- ❀ 2 pounds Italian sausage links, cut into 2-inch pieces
- ❀ 1/4 cup olive oil
- ❀ 4 large potatoes, peeled and thickly sliced
- ❀ 2 large green bell peppers, seeded and cut into wedges
- ❀ 2 large red bell peppers, seeded and cut into wedges
- ❀ 3 large onions, cut into wedges
- ❀ 1/2 cup white wine
- ❀ 1/2 cup chicken stock
- ❀ 1 teaspoon Italian seasoning salt and pepper to taste

Directions

- ➢ Preheat oven to 400 degrees F (200 degrees C).Heat 2 teaspoons olive oil in a large skillet over medium heat, and cook and stir the sausage until browned. Transfer the cooked sausage to a large baking dish.

- ➢ Pour 1/4 cup of olive oil into the skillet, and cook the potatoes, stirring occasionally, until browned, about 10 minutes.

- ➢ Place the potatoes into the baking dish, leaving some oil. Cook and stir the green and red peppers and onions in the hot skillet until they are beginning to soften, about 5 minutes.

- ➢ Add the vegetables to the baking dish. Pour wine and chicken stock over the vegetables and sausage, and sprinkle with Italian seasoning, salt, and pepper.

- ➢ Gently stir the sausage, potatoes, and vegetables together.Bake in the preheated oven until hot and bubbling, 20 to 25 minutes. Serve hot.

Country Scalloped Potatoes

Ingredients

- 1 (10.75 ounce) can Campbell's® Condensed Cream of Celery Soup (Regular or 98% Fat Free)
- 1 (10.5 ounce) can Campbell's® Chicken Gravy
- 1 cup milk
- 5 medium baking potatoes, peeled and thinly sliced
- 1 small onion, thinly sliced
- 2 1/2 cups diced cooked ham
- 1 cup shredded Cheddar cheese

Directions

- Stir soup, gravy and milk in bowl. Layer half the potatoes, onion, ham and soup mixture in 13x9x2" shallow baking dish. Repeat layers. Cover.

- Bake at 375 degrees F for 40 minutes. Uncover and bake 25 minutes. Top with cheese. Bake 5 minutes more or until potatoes are tender and cheese melts. Let stand 10 minutes.

Sweet Potatoes with Brandy and Raisins

Ingredients

- ❋ 1/4 cup brandy
- ❋ 1/2 cup raisins
- ❋ 2 tablespoons softened butter
- ❋ 4 (1 pound) sweet potatoes
- ❋ 1/4 cup packed brown sugar

Directions

➢ Pour brandy over raisins in a small bowl, cover, and allow to stand for 2 hours. Preheat oven to 350 degrees F (175 degrees C). Butter a 2-quart baking dish with the softened butter.

➢ Place sweet potatoes on a baking sheet, and bake in preheated oven until tender, about 30 minutes. Remove and allow to cool until cool enough to handle, then peel the potatoes and slice them 1/2 inch thick.

➢ Arrange the potato slices in the prepared baking dish, and sprinkle with sugar and brandy-soaked raisins. Return the sweet potatoes to the oven, and bake 30 to 40 minutes until hot and bubbly.

Potatoes and Corn Soup

Ingredients

- 6 medium potatoes, peeled and cubed
- 6 stalks celery, chopped, leaves reserved
- 1 medium onion, chopped
- 2 cubes chicken bouillon
- 2 (15.25 ounce) cans whole kernel corn, drained
- 1/4 cup chopped fresh chives

Directions

- In a large pot, place the potatoes, celery and leaves, and onion. Pour in enough water to cover. Bring to a boil. Remove the celery leaves, and stir in the bouillon cubes until dissolved. Mix in the corn.

- Reduce heat to medium-low, and cook 20 minutes, or until the potatoes are tender. Mix the chives into the pot, and continue cooking 5 minutes before serving.

Colleen's Potato Crescent Rolls

Ingredients

- 2 potatoes, peeled and cut into 1 inch cubes
- 1 (.25 ounce) package active dry yeast
- 1 1/2 cups warm water (110 degrees F/45 degrees C)
- 2/3 cup white sugar
- 2/3 cup shortening
- 2 eggs
- 1 1/2 teaspoons salt
- 6 1/2 cups all-purpose flour
- 1/4 cup butter, melted

Directions

➢ Place potatoes in a saucepan, and cover with water. Bring to a boil, and cook until tender, about 15 minutes. Drain, cool, and mash.

➢ In a large bowl, dissolve yeast in warm water. Let stand until creamy, about 10 minutes.

➢ When yeast is ready, mix in 1 cup mashed potatoes, sugar, shortening, eggs, salt, and 3 cups flour. Stir in the remaining flour, 1/2 cup at a time, until dough has become stiff but still pliable.

➢ Turn dough out onto a lightly floured surface, and knead until smooth and elastic, about 8 minutes. Lightly oil a large bowl, place the dough in the bowl, and turn to coat with oil. Cover with plastic wrap, and refrigerate for at least 8 hours, and up to 5 days.

➢ Deflate the dough, and turn it out onto a lightly floured surface. Divide the dough into two equal pieces, and form into rounds. Roll out each round to a 12 inch circle. Brush generously with melted butter, and cut each circle into 16 wedges.

➢ Roll wedges up tightly, starting with the large end. Place on lightly greased baking sheets with the points underneath, and the ends bent to form a crescent shape.

➢ Cover, and let rise for 1 hour. Meanwhile, preheat oven to 400 degrees F (200 degrees C).Bake in preheated oven for 15 to 20 minutes, or until golden

Potato Soup I

Ingredients

- 6 potatoes, peeled and cubed
- 1 onion, chopped
- 1 carrot, grated
- 4 slices crisp cooked bacon, crumbled
- salt to taste
- ground black pepper to taste
- 1 tablespoon chopped fresh parsley
- 1 tablespoon margarine
- 1 tablespoon rendered bacon fat
- 4 cups milk
- 3 tablespoons dry potato flakes

Directions

➢ Place potatoes and chopped onion in a deep stock pan, and add water just to cover them. Bring to a boil, and cook until tender.

➢ Add butter or margarine, bacon bits and fat, and carrots. Stir in milk, parsley, and instant potatoes; bring to a light boil. Salt and pepper to taste. Cover, and simmer on low until you are ready to eat.

Ellen Szaller's Mashed Potato Pancakes

Ingredients

- 2 cups sifted all-purpose flour
- 1 teaspoon salt
- 1 tablespoon baking powder
- 3 potatoes - peeled, boiled and mashed
- 1 onion, chopped
- 2 eggs
- 1 cup milk
- 1/4 cup light corn syrup
- 1 teaspoon ground nutmeg
- 2 tablespoons shortening

Directions

➢ In a medium bowl, mix together flour, salt, and baking powder. Stir in mashed potatoes and onion until thoroughly combined. In a separate bowl, whisk together eggs and milk, and stir lightly into potato mixture.

➢ Stir in corn syrup and nutmeg, mixing well. Heat a large griddle to medium-high heat. Coat with shortening and spoon potato mixture onto griddle in 12 equal portions. Fry until brown on both sides. Serve hot.

Easy Cheesy Scalloped Potatoes

Ingredients

- 1 (8 ounce) package
- PHILADELPHIA Cream Cheese, softened
- 1/2 cup KNUDSEN Sour Cream
- 1 cup chicken broth
- 3 pounds red potatoes, thinly sliced
- 1 (6 ounce) package sliced ham, chopped
- 1 (8 ounce) package shredded Cheddar cheese, divided
- 1 cup frozen peas

Directions

> Heat oven to 350 degrees F. Mix cream cheese, sour cream and broth in large bowl until well blended. Add potatoes, ham, 1-3/4 cups of the cheese and peas; stir gently to coat all ingredients.

> Spoon into 13x9-inch baking dish sprayed with cooking spray. Sprinkle with remaining cheese.Bake 1 hour or until casserole is heated through and potatoes are tender.

Easy Spicy Roasted Potatoes

Ingredients

- 5 medium red potatoes, diced with peel
- 1 medium onion, chopped
- 1 tablespoon garlic powder
- 1 tablespoon kosher salt
- 2 teaspoons chili powder
- 1/4 cup extra virgin olive oil
- 1 cup shredded Cheddar cheese (optional)

Directions

➤ Preheat the oven to 450 degrees F (220 degrees C). Arrange the potatoes and onions in a greased 9x13 inch baking dish so that they are evenly distributed.

➤ Season with garlic powder, salt and chili powder. Drizzle with olive oil. Stir to coat potatoes and onions with oil and spices.

➤ Bake for 35 to 40 minutes in the preheated oven, until potatoes are fork tender and slightly crispy.

➤ Stir every 10 minutes. When done, sprinkle with cheese. Wait about 5 minutes for the cheese to melt before serving.

Roasted Sweet Potato and Carrot Puree

Ingredients

- ❉ 1 pound sweet potatoes, peeled, cut into 1/2 inch pieces
- ❉ 8 carrots, peeled, cut into 1/2-inch slices
- ❉ 3 tablespoons olive oil
- ❉ 2 tablespoons brown sugar
- ❉ 1 teaspoon salt
- ❉ 1 1/2 cups chicken broth, divided
- ❉ 4 ounces PHILADELPHIA Cream Cheese, cubed

Directions

➢ Heat oven to 375 degrees F. Combine first 5 ingredients; spread onto bottom of 15x10x1-inch pan. Pour 1 cup broth over vegetable mixture.

➢ Bake 45 to 55 min. or until broth is absorbed and vegetables are tender and caramelized, stirring occasionally.

➢ Spoon vegetables into food processor. Add cream cheese and remaining broth; process until smooth. Return to pan; cook until heated through, stirring frequently.

Cream Cheese Ranch Potatoes

Ingredients

- 8 baking potatoes, peeled and quartered
- 1 (8 ounce) package cream cheese, softened
- 1 (1 ounce) package dry Ranch-style dressing mix
- 1 cup sour cream
- 1/2 cup butter, softened

Directions

➤ Bring a large pot of salted water to a boil. Add potatoes and cook until tender, about 25 minutes. Drain and mash.

➤ In a large bowl beat the cream cheese and dressing mix until smooth. Stir in mashed potatoes, sour cream and butter; beat until desired consistency is reached.

Potato Salad with Bacon, Olives, and Radishes

Ingredients

- 5 potatoes
- 1 pound bacon
- 2 stalks celery
- 4 small green onions
- 12 stuffed green olives
- 5 radishes
- 1/4 cup mayonnaise
- 1 tablespoon lemon juice

Directions

➢ Wash and peel the potatoes and cut into 1/2 to 3/4 inch pieces. Bring a large pot of salted water to a boil. Add the potatoes and cook until tender but still firm, about 10 minutes.

➢ Slice the bacon into small pieces and cook over medium high heat in a large, deep skillet until evenly brown. Do not overcook.

➢ Chop the celery, green onions, stuffed olives and radishes into small pieces and put into a large bowl. Add the potatoes and bacon and mix together.

➢ Add the mayonnaise and lemon juice to taste, stir, and place in the refrigerator for a few hours to chill before serving. You may want to add a few sliced hard boiled eggs on top. ENJOY!!!

Cheesy Rosemary Potatoes

Ingredients

- 1 medium onion, thinly sliced
- 3 cloves garlic, minced
- 1 tablespoon olive or vegetable oil
- 4 large potatoes, peeled and diced
- 1 teaspoon seasoned salt
- 1/8 teaspoon pepper
- 1/2 teaspoon grated lemon peel
- 2 cups shredded Cheddar cheese, divided
- 1/4 cup dry bread crumbs
- 1 tablespoon butter or margarine, melted
- 1/2 teaspoon dried rosemary, crushed

Directions

➢ In a large skillet or saucepan, saute onion and garlic in oil until tender. Add potatoes, seasoned salt, pepper and lemon peel.

➢ Remove from the heat. Spoon half into a greased 1-1/2-qt. baking dish. Sprinkle with 1 cup cheese. Repeat layers.

➢ Combine bread crumbs, butter and rosemary; sprinkle over cheese. Cover and bake at 400 degrees F for 40 minutes. Uncover and bake 20 minutes longer or until potatoes are tender.

Bob Evans® Au Gratin Potatoes

Ingredients

- ❀ 1 (20 ounce) package Bob Evans® Hash Brown Potatoes
- ❀ 1 tablespoon flour
- ❀ 1/2 teaspoon salt
- ❀ 1/4 teaspoon pepper
- ❀ 1/4 teaspoon onion powder
- ❀ 2 cups shredded Cheddar cheese, divided
- ❀ 2 tablespoons shredded Parmesan cheese
- ❀ 1 cup milk
- ❀ 2 tablespoons butter or margarine, melted

Directions

➢ Preheat oven to 350 degrees F. Grease 9x9 inch baking pan. Blend together flour, salt, pepper and onion powder. Set aside.

➢ In a large bowl combine Bob Evans hash brown potatoes and dry seasoning mixture, mix together. Place half of potato mixture into baking pan. Top with 1 cup of cheddar cheese.

➢ Place other half of potato mixture on top and top with 1 cup of cheddar cheese and parmesan cheese.

➢ Pour milk and melted butter or margarine over mixture. Bake for 45-50 minutes or until top is golden brown.

Apple Cider Sweet Potatoes

Ingredients

- 3 pounds sweet potatoes, peeled and cubed
- 1 cup apple cider
- 1/2 teaspoon salt
- 1 tablespoon butter
- 1 pinch ground black pepper

Directions

- Combine the sweet potatoes, apple cider, and salt in a large pot over high heat. Bring to a boil.

- Reduce heat, cover and simmer until potatoes are tender, 20 to 30 minutes. Mash potatoes together with the cider until smooth. Stir in the butter, and season with pepper.

Scalloped Potato-Onion Bake

Ingredients

- Condensed Cream of Celery Soup (Regular or 98% Fat Free)
- 1/2 cup milk
- 1 dash ground black pepper
- 4 medium potatoes, thinly sliced
- 1 small onion, thinly sliced
- 1 tablespoon butter, cut into small pieces
- Paprika
- 1 (10.75 ounce) can Campbell's®

Directions

- Stir the soup, milk and black pepper in a small bowl. Layer half the potatoes, onion and soup mixture in a 1 1/2-quart casserole.

- Repeat the layers. Dot the top with the butter. Sprinkle with the paprika. Cover the baking dish.

- Bake at 400 degrees F for 1 hour. Uncover the dish and bake for 15 minutes or until the potatoes are tender.

Potato Bacon Chowder

Ingredients

- 2 cups peeled, cubed potatoes
- 1 cup water
- 8 bacon strips
- 1 cup chopped onion
- 1/2 cup chopped celery
- 1 (10.75 ounce) can condensed cream of chicken soup, undiluted
- 1 3/4 cups milk
- 1 cup sour cream
- 1/2 teaspoon salt Dash pepper
- 1 tablespoon minced fresh parsley

Directions

➢ In a covered 3-qt. saucepan, cook potatoes in water until tender. Meanwhile, cook bacon in a skillet until crisp; remove to paper towels to drain.

➢ In the same skillet, saute onion and celery in drippings until tender; drain. Add to undrained potatoes. Stir in soup, milk, sour cream, salt and pepper. Cook over low heat for 10 minutes or until heated through (do not boil).

➢ Crumble bacon; set aside 1/4 cup. Add remaining bacon to soup along with parsley. Sprinkle with reserved bacon.

Hasselback Potatoes

Ingredients

- ❀ 4 (8 ounce) baking potatoes
- ❀ 2 tablespoons butter, melted salt and pepper to taste
- ❀ 2 tablespoons finely grated fresh Romano cheese
- ❀ 1 tablespoon seasoned dry bread crumbs

Directions

➤ Preheat the oven to 425 degrees F (220 degrees C). Peel the potatoes, and place in bowl of cold water to prevent browning. Place potatoes into a large wooden or metal spoon.

➤ Using a sharp knife, make slices across the potato the short way about 1/8 to 1/4 inch apart, making sure to cut down to the lip of the spoon, not all the way through the potato.

➤ The slices should stay connected at the bottom, and the spoon helps keep the depth even. Return the potato to the bowl of water, and proceed with the remaining potatoes.

➤ When all of the potatoes are cut, place them cut side up in a shallow baking dish or small roasting pan. Drizzle with half of the butter, then season with salt and pepper.

➤ Bake for 35 to 40 minutes in the preheated oven. Remove from the oven, and drizzle with the remaining butter.

➤ Sprinkle Romano cheese and bread crumbs onto the tops of the potatoes, and season with a little more salt and pepper. Return to the oven, and bake for an additional 20 minutes, or until nicely browned.

Sweet Potato Casserole IV

Ingredients

* 3 cups cooked and mashed sweet potatoes
* 1 cup white sugar
* 1/2 cup butter
* 1/3 cup evaporated milk
* 2 eggs, beaten
* 1 teaspoon vanilla extract
* 1/3 cup butter, melted
* 1 cup chopped pecans
* 1 cup packed light brown sugar 1/2 cup all-purpose flour

Directions

➢ Mix together sweet potatoes, white sugar, 1/2 cup butter or margarine, milk, eggs, and vanilla. Spread into a greased 9 x 13 inch baking dish.

➢ Mix together 1/3 cup melted butter or marg-arine, pecans,brown sug-ar, and flour. Spoon on top of sweet potato mixture.Bake at 350 degrees F (175 degrees C) for 25 to 30 minutes.

Alfredo Potatoes

Ingredients

- 2 large baking potatoes
- 1 cup prepared Alfredo sauce
- 1 teaspoon garlic powder
- 1/2 teaspoon pepper
- 1/8 teaspoon dried thyme
- 1 cup shredded Cheddar cheese, divided
- 1/2 cup shredded mozzarella cheese

Directions

- Pierce potatoes several times with a fork and place on a microwave-safe plate. Microwave on high for 6 minutes or until tender. Allow potatoes to cool slightly.

- Meanwhile, in a bowl, combine the Alfredo sauce, garlic powder, pepper and thyme. Stir in 1/2 cup cheddar cheese and mozzarella cheese. Cut potatoes in half lengthwise.

- Scoop out the pulp and add to the sauce mixture; mix well. Spoon into potato shells.Sprinkle with remaining cheddar cheese. Microwave on high for 1 minute or until cheese is melted.

Potato **Lasagna**

Ingredients

- ❋ 10 small red potatoes, thinly sliced
- ❋ 10 baby carrots, sliced
- ❋ 1 large green bell pepper, chopped
- ❋ 1/2 Vidalia onion, chopped
- ❋ 3 cloves garlic, chopped
- ❋ 2 cups baby spinach leaves
- ❋ 1/4 cup shredded smoked Gouda cheese
- ❋ 1 1/2 cups shredded mozzarella cheese
- ❋ 1/2 cup shredded sharp Cheddar cheese
- ❋ salt and pepper to taste
- ❋ 1 (14 ounce) jar vodka marinara sauce

Directions

- ➢ Preheat the oven to 350 degrees F (175 degrees C). Lightly grease a 2 quart casserole dish.

- ➢ In a medium bowl, toss together the carrots, bell pepper, onion, garlic, and spinach. In a separate bowl, blend together the Gouda cheese, mozzarella cheese, and sharp Cheddar cheese. Set aside.

- ➢ Place two layers of sliced potatoes in the bottom of the prepared casserole dish. Season the potatoes with a little salt and pepper. Top with a layer of the spinach mixture, and pour about 1/2 cup of sauce over all.

- ➢ Sprinkle with some of the cheese blend. Repeat layering with remaining potatoes, vege-tables, sauce and cheese, ending with cheese on the top.

- ➢ Bake covered for 35 minutes in the preheated oven. Remove the lid, and bake for 10 more minutes until the top is browned.

Potato Soup IV

Ingredients

- 2 tablespoons margarine
- 1/3 cup chopped celery
- 1/3 cup chopped onion
- 6 cups peeled and diced red potatoes
- 4 cups chicken broth
- 4 cups milk
- 1 1/2 teaspoons salt
- 1/4 teaspoon ground black pepper
- 1 tablespoon cornstarch
- 1/4 cup water
- 2 cups shredded sharp Cheddar cheese

Directions

➤ In large saucepan, heat butter or margarine over medium heat. Add celery and onions; cook and stir until tender.

➤ Add potatoes and broth, and simmer until tender. Stir in milk, and season with salt and pepper. Dissolve cornstarch in 1/4 cup water, and slowly stir into soup.

➤ Bring to a boil for 1 minute, and then turn heat to medium-low. Stir in 2 cups cheese, and continue stirring until it melts. Serve.

Scalloped Potatoes

Ingredients

- 5 potatoes, peeled and sliced
- 1 (8 ounce) package Cheddar cheese, cubed
- 1/2 cup butter
- 1 cup milk
- 2 teaspoons cooking sherry
- 1 cup cornflakes cereal crumbs

Directions

- Preheat oven to 350 degrees F (175 degrees C). Bring a large pot of salted water to a boil. Add potatoes and cook until tender, about 15 minutes. Drain and place in a 2 quart casserole dish.

- In a microwave safe dish combine cheese, butter and milk. Microwave until cheese and butter melt; stir in the sherry.

- Pour cheese mixture over potatoes and sprinkle corn-flakes crumbs on top. Bake in preheated oven for 15 to 30 minutes, or until heated through.

Cheddar Potato Bake

Ingredients

* 3 cups mashed potatoes*
* 1 (10.75 ounce) can Campbell's® Condensed Cheddar Cheese
* Soup
* 1/3 cup sour cream or yogurt Generous dash ground black pepper
* 1 green onion, chopped

'Directions

➢ Stir the potatoes, soup, sour cream, black pepper and onion in a medium bowl. Spoon into a 1 1/2-quart baking dish.

➢ Bake at 350 degrees F for 30 minutes or until the potato mixture is hot.

Red Potato Salad with Sour Cream and Chives

Ingredients

- 6 large red potatoes
- 1/2 cup sour cream
- 1/2 cup plain yogurt
- 1/4 cup fresh chives, finely chopped
- 1 teaspoon salt ground black pepper to taste

Directions

➤ Scrub potatoes (don't peel). If large, cut in half or in quarters. Boil potatoes in their skins until fork-tender. Drain, dry and cut into 1/2 inch cubes.

➤ In a salad bowl, combine the potatoes, sour cream, yogurt, and chives; toss gently to coat. Add salt, and pepper to taste; refrigerate until chilled.

Herbed New Potatoes

Ingredients

- 3/4 pound small red potatoes
- 1 tablespoon butter, softened
- 1 tablespoon sour cream
- 2 teaspoons snipped fresh dill
- 2 teaspoons minced chives
- 1/4 teaspoon salt
- 1/8 teaspoon pepper
- 1 dash lemon juice

Directions

➤ Remove a strip of peel from the middle of each potato. Place potatoes in a saucepan and cover with water. Bring to a boil over medium heat. Reduce heat; cover and simmer for 20 minutes or until tender.

➤ In a small bowl, combine the remaining ingredients. Drain potatoes; add butter mixture and toss gently.

Brilliant Potatoes With Paprika and Caramelized

Ingredients

- ❀ 3 tablespoons canola oil
- ❀ 2 large Vidalia or other sweet onions, roughly chopped
- ❀ 4 (15 ounce) cans whole new potatoes, drained
- ❀ 3 tablespoons extra-virgin olive oil
- ❀ 3/4 teaspoon garlic salt
- ❀ 1/4 teaspoon garlic powder
- ❀ 1/4 teaspoon dried minced garlic
- ❀ 2 tablespoons paprika
- ❀ 1/4 teaspoon black pepper
- ❀ 1/2 cup butter, at room temperature

Directions

➤ Preheat oven to 400 degrees F (200 degrees C). Grease a 9x13 inch baking dish. Heat the canola oil in a large skillet over medium heat, then stir in the Vidalia onion.

➤ Cook and stir until the onion has softened and turned deep brown, 10 to 15 minutes. While the onions are caramelizing, toss the drained potatoes with the olive oil in a large bowl.

➤ Season with garlic salt, garlic powder, dried minced garlic, and black pepper; toss until well coated, then pour into the prepared baking dish, and spread into a single layer.

➤ Sprinkle the caramelized onions on top of the potatoes, then dot the top of the dish with the room temperature butter, and sprinkle with paprika. Bake uncovered in the preheated oven until the outsides of the potatoes are crisp, 45 to 55 minutes.

Sweet Potato Chimichangas

Ingredients

- 1 (40 ounce) can mashed sweet potatoes
- 1 tablespoon ground cinnamon
- 1 (10 ounce) package miniature marshmallows
- 1 tablespoon frozen whipped topping, thawed
- 1/2 cup confectioners' sugar
- 1/3 cup all-purpose flour
- 16 (10 inch) flour tortillas
- 1/4 cup butter, softened
- 1 quart oil for frying, or as needed
- 1 1/2 teaspoons ground cinnamon
- 1 tablespoon white sugar

Directions

- Place the sweet potatoes in a saucepan, and stir in 1 tablespoon of cinnamon. Cook and stir over medium heat until most of the juice has evaporated. Stir in the marshmallows just until partly melted. Remove from heat, and set aside to cool.

- Once the sweet potato mixture is cool, stir in the confectioners' sugar and flour. Add more sugar to taste if desired.

- Cut each tortilla in half, and spread a thin layer of butter on each side. Place 1 tablespoon of the sweet potato filling onto the center of each one running parallel to the cut edge, then fold in the sides, and roll up from the straight edge to seal in the filling.

- Heat about 1 inch oil in a large heavy skillet to about 350 degrees F (175 degrees C). Fry chimichangas until light golden brown, turning as needed.

- Remove to paper towels to drain. The tortillas will darken a little after they are removed. Mix together the remaining cinnamon and sugar. Sprinkle over the chimichangas while warm.

Sweet Potato Balls

Ingredients

- 40 ounces canned sweet potatoes
- 1/4 cup butter
- 1 pinch salt (optional)
- 3 cups crushed cornflakes cereal
- 3/4 cup real maple syrup
- 10 large marshmallows

Directions

➢ Drain sweet potatoes and put into large mixing bowl. Mash the potatoes with butter or margarine. Salt to tate.

➢ Hand pat mixture into 3 inch diameter balls. Roll in crushed corn flakes and put into 9 x 12 inch greased baking dish. Pour maple syrup evenly over all balls.

➢ Bake at 325 degrees F (165 degrees C) for 40 minutes. The last fifteen minutes put a marshmallow over each ball.

Potato Salad Soup

Ingredients

- 5 tablespoons unsalted butter
- 1 onion, chopped
- 1/2 cup chopped celery
- 1/4 cup chopped carrots
- 2 cloves garlic, minced
- 2 tablespoons chopped fresh parsley
- 4 tablespoons all-purpose flour
- 1 1/2 cups chicken stock
- 1 1/2 cups milk
- 3 potatoes, cut into 1/4-inch slices
- 2 teaspoons Worcestershire sauce
- 1 1/2 teaspoons mustard powder
- 1 pinch ground allspice
- 3/4 teaspoon celery salt
- 1/2 teaspoon dried thyme
- 1/2 teaspoon seasoning salt
- 2 tablespoons white wine
- 1/4 teaspoon poultry seasoning
- 3 hard-cooked eggs, chopped

Directions

- Saute the onion, celery, carrots, garlic, and parsley in the butter until soft. Sprinkle in the flour and cook, stirring, for 2 minutes.

- Add the stock, milk, potatoes, Worcestershire sauce, dry mustard powder, allspice, celery salt, thyme, seasoning salt, white wine and poultry seasoning. Allow to simmer and thicken, stirring occasionally.

- Cook until the potatoes are cooked through, about 25 minutes. During the cook-ing break up the potatoes with the back of a spoon to make large chunks. Serve warm with chopped hard boiled egg sprinkled over.

PJ's Sweet Potato Mash

Ingredients

- 6 (8 ounce) sweet potatoes
- 1 1/2 tablespoons prepared horseradish
- 2 tablespoons honey
- 2 tablespoons butter or margarine
- 1/2 teaspoon salt
- 1/4 cup heavy cream

Directions

- ➤ Preheat the oven to 400 degrees F (200 degrees C). Place potatoes on a baking sheet and bake for 40 to 50 minutes, until tenderenough to easily pierce with a fork. Cool slightly and remove peels.

- ➤ Place the cooked sweet potatoes into a large bowl and mash with the horseradish, honey, butter and salt.

- ➤ Whip with an electric mixer until light and fluffy, adding heavy cream as needed to get the texture you desire. Serve immediately, or keep warm in the oven until time to serve.

White Potato Dressing

Ingredients

- 10 pounds white potatoes, peeled and quartered
- 1 pound spicy Italian sausage, casing removed
- 1 red bell pepper, chopped
- 1 onion, chopped
- 2 (8 ounce) cans tomato sauce
- 1/2 pound raisins
- 1 pinch dried sage
- 1 pinch garlic powder
- salt and pepper to taste

Directions

- Preheat oven to 350 degrees F (175 degrees C). Grease two 9x12 inch baking dishes. Place sausage in a large, deep skillet.

- Crumble and cook over medium high heat. Add bell pepper and onion to sausage and cook until sausage is evenly brown.

- Bring a pot of salted water to a boil. Add potatoes; cook until tender but still firm. Drain, and transfer to a large bowl.

- Mash potatoes until smooth and add to sausage mixture. Stir in tomato sauce, raisins, sage, garlic powder, salt and pepper. Pour into baking dishes and bake for 25 to 35 minutes.

Garlic Baked Potato

Ingredients

- 4 medium baking potatoes, scrubbed
- 2 tablespoons olive oil
- 2 teaspoons garlic salt, or to taste
- salt and pepper to taste

Directions

- ➢ Preheat the oven to 375 degrees F (190 degrees C). Pour olive oil into a plastic bag. Measure the garlic salt and pepper onto a plate, and stir around a little. Coat each potato with olive oil by placing in the bag, and moving it around.

- ➢ Remove from the bag, and dip into the seasoning. Rub seasoning into the potato to coat. Place the potatoes directly on the oven rack. Bake for 1 hour in the preheated oven, or until the potatoes feel soft when you squeeze them.

Crawfish Potato Soup

Ingredients

- 3 slices bacon
- 1 onion, chopped
- 1 green bell pepper, seeded and chopped
- 1 red bell pepper, seeded and chopped
- 2 stalks celery, finely chopped
- 2 tablespoons minced garlic
- 5 cups diced red potatoes
- 1 cup grated carrot
- 1 pound crawfish tails
- 3 cups chicken broth
- 1 quart half-and-half cream salt and pepper to taste
- 1 cup shredded Cheddar cheese

Directions

➤ Place the bacon into a large pot over medium-high heat. Cook until crisp, turning as needed. Crumble, and return to the pot.

➤ Reduce the heat to medium, and add the onion, green pepper, red pepper, celery. and garlic. Cook and stir until the onion is transparent, and the peppers are soft.

➤ Add the crawfish, and cook until the liquid evaporates, and the crawfish begin to brown. Remove the contents of the pot, and set aside.

➤ Pour the chicken broth into the pot, and add the potatoes. If the chicken broth does not cover the potatoes, add enough water to compensate.

➤ Bring to a boil, and cook for 8 to 10 minutes, or until the potatoes are soft. Add the carrots, and cook for about 8 more minutes.

➤ Reduce the heat to low, and return the vegetables and crawfish to the pot. Stir in the half-and-half, and heat through. Do not boil.Season with salt and pepper to taste. Ladle into bowls and garnish with Cheddar cheese to serve.

Rich Mashed Potatoes

Ingredients

* 5 pounds potatoes - peeled and cubed
* 5 tablespoons butter or margarine, divided
* 1 (8 ounce) package cream cheese, cubed
* 1 cup sour cream
* 2 teaspoons onion salt 1/4 teaspoon garlic powder
* 1/4 teaspoon pepper

Directions

> Cook potatoes in boiling salted water until very tender, about 20-25 minutes; drain well. Mash with 3 tablespoons of butter.

> Add cream cheese, sour cream, onion salt, garlic powder and pepper; mix well. Spoon into a greased 13-in. x 9-in. x 2-in. baking dish.

> Melt remaining butter; drizzle over the top. Cover and freeze for up to 1 month. Or bake,uncovered, at 350 degrees for 30-35 minutes or until heated through.

> To use frozen potatoes: Thaw in the refrigerator. Bake as directed.

Sweet Potato Pineapple Casserole

Ingredients

- 3 sweet potatoes
- 1/2 cup crushed pineapple with juice
- 1/4 cup packed light brown sugar
- 3 tablespoons butter

Directions

➢ Preheat oven to 350 degrees F (175 degrees C). Lightly grease a 9x13 inch baking dish. In a large soup pot, boil sweet potatoes whole until soft.

➢ Remove skins, and dice into bite-sized pieces. Mix sweet potatoes, crushed pineapple, light brown sugar, and butter in prepared baking dish. Bake for 45 minutes, or until casserole is mushy with no excess water in the dish.

Grandma Sophie's Smashed Potato Salad

Ingredients

- 5 pounds potatoes, peeled, cut into 2 inch chunks
- 3 hard-cooked eggs, peeled and finely diced
- 1/2 cup finely chopped dill pickle
- 2 cups mayonnaise
- salt to taste

Directions

➤ Boil potatoes until soft, about 25 to 30 minutes. Remove potatoes to a large bowl.While the potatoes are still warm but not steaming, stir in the hard-cooked eggs with a fork.

➤ Mix in the dill pickle, then stir in the mayonnaise. Season to taste with salt. Continue to stir until potatoes are smashed and not many big chunks remain.

Candie's Easy Potato and Onion Dish

Ingredients

- 8 potatoes, sliced
- 2 large sweet onions, sliced
- 1/2 cup butter, sliced
- 1 tablespoon dried parsley
- salt and pepper to taste

Directions

- Preheat oven to 350 degrees F (175 degrees C). In a 9x13 inch casserole dish, mix the potatoes, onions, butter, and parsley. Season with salt and pepper.

- Bake covered in the preheated oven for 45 minutes, stirring occasion-nally, or until potatoes are tender.

Raisin Sweet Potato Bread

Ingredients

- 2 cups self-rising flour*
- 2 cups sugar
- 3 teaspoons ground cinnamon
- 1/2 teaspoon ground nutmeg
- 1/4 teaspoon ground cloves
- 1 1/2 cups mashed cooked sweet potatoes
- 1 cup vegetable oil
- 3 eggs
- 3 teaspoons vanilla extract
- 3/4 cup raisins

Directions

- In a bowl, combine the flour, sugar, cinnamon, nutmeg and cloves. Combine the sweet potatoes, oil, eggs and vanilla; stir into the dry ingredients just until moistened.

- Fold in raisins. Transfer to two greased 8-in. x 4-in. x 2-in. loaf pans. Bake at 350 degrees F for 55 -60 minutes or until a toothpick inserted near the center comes out clean. Cool for 10 minutes before removing from pans to wire racks.

Cheesy Broccoli Potato Topper

Ingredients

- 4 hot baked potatoes, split
- 1 cup cooked broccoli flowerets
- 1 (10.75 ounce) can Campbell's® Condensed Cheddar Cheese Soup

Directions

> Place the potatoes onto a microwavable plate. Top with the broccoli. Spoon the soup over the broccoli. Microwave on HIGH for 4 minutes or until the soup is hot.

Potato Soup

Ingredients

- 1 tablespoon butter
- 1 large onion, chopped
- 6 cups mashed cooked potatoes
- 2 (14.5 ounce) cans chicken broth
- 1/2 cup milk

Directions

> In a medium soup pot melt butter over low heat, and saute onions until tender. Stir in the mashed potatoes, and then slowly add the chicken broth.

> Stirring, add milk (use more or less to achieve desired creami-ness). Cook until heated through and season with salt and pepper to taste.

Potato Soup Italian Style

Ingredients

- ❀ 3 tablespoons olive oil
- ❀ 1 large onion, chopped
- ❀ 5 cups water
- ❀ 4 potatoes, peeled and quartered
- ❀ salt and pepper to taste
- ❀ 4 eggs

Directions

➢ Heat oil in a large pot over medium heat. Saute onions until translucent. To the onions add water, potatoes, salt and pepper. Bring to a boil; reduce heat to low and simmer for 20 minutes, or until potatoes are tender but still firm.

➢ Remove from heat and gently crack eggs into soup; be careful not to break eggs. Place on low heat until whites of eggs are cooked. Cool slightly before serving.

Lightning Source UK Ltd.
Milton Keynes UK
UKHW050632010621
384722UK00002B/195

9 781803 015569